When Someone You K

A JOHNS HOPKINS PRESS HEALTH BOOK

When Someone You Know
Has DEPRESSION

Words to Say and Things to Do

Susan J. Noonan, MD, MPH

Foreword by Timothy J. Petersen, PhD,

Jonathan E. Alpert, MD, PhD,

and Andrew A. Nierenberg, MD

JOHNS HOPKINS UNIVERSITY PRESS

Baltimore

Note to the reader: This book is not meant to substitute for medical care of people who have depression or other mental disorders, and treatment should not be based solely on its contents. Instead, treatment must be developed in a dialogue between the individual and his or her physician. My book has been written to help with that dialogue.

If you or someone you know is thinking about suicide, immediately contact your health care provider, go to the nearest Emergency Department, or call 9-1-1.

© 2016 Johns Hopkins University Press
All rights reserved. Published 2016
Printed in the United States of America on acid-free paper
9 8 7 6 5 4 3 2 1

Johns Hopkins University Press
2715 North Charles Street
Baltimore, Maryland 21218-4363
www.press.jhu.edu

Library of Congress Cataloging-in-Publication Data

Names: Noonan, Susan J., 1953– author.
Title: When someone you know has depression : words to say and things to do /
    Susan J. Noonan, MD, MPH ; foreword by Timothy J. Petersen, PhD, Jonathan E. Alpert,
    MD, PhD, and Andrew A. Nierenberg, MD.
Description: Baltimore : Johns Hopkins University Press, 2016. | Series: A Johns Hopkins
    Press health book | Includes bibliographical references and index.
Identifiers: LCCN 2015035546| ISBN 9781421420141 (hardcover) | ISBN 1421420147
    (hardcover) | ISBN 9781421420158 (paperback) | ISBN 1421420155 (paperback)
    | ISBN 9781421420165 (electronic) | ISBN 1421420163 (electronic)
Subjects: LCSH: Depression, Mental—Popular works. | Self-care, Health—Popular works.
    | BISAC: SELF-HELP / Depression. | PSYCHOLOGY / Psychopathology / Depression.
    | MEDICAL / Public Health.
Classification: LCC RC537 .N663 2016 | DDC 616.85/27—dc23 LC record available at
    http://lccn.loc.gov/2015035546

A catalog record for this book is available from the British Library.

Special discounts are available for bulk purchases of this book. For more information, please contact Special Sales at 410-516-6936 or specialsales@press.jhu.edu.

Johns Hopkins University Press uses environmentally friendly book materials, including recycled text paper that is composed of at least 30 percent postconsumer waste, whenever possible.

Contents

Charts and Tables

Charts

Tables

Foreword

It is our privilege to write the foreword to Dr. Noonan's book *When Someone You Know Has Depression: Words to Say and Things to Do.* Depression affects not only millions of people each year, but also their close relationships. When depressed, individuals may be more distant, sensitive, or irritable around loved ones. In turn, family members or friends may respond by "trying too hard to help" or, alternatively, by distancing themselves. A downward spiral can result in which depressed individuals begin to view themselves as less capable and worthy of being cared for, while their loved ones may feel sad, powerless, frustrated, desperate, and sometimes burned out. Even the most caring individuals can feel they are "walking on eggshells" around a loved one who is depressed and can feel at a loss to know how to help.

When Someone You Know Has Depression is a thoughtful and perfect companion to Dr. Noonan's first book, *Managing Your Depression.* While that book provides valuable information and skills to those suffering with depression, this book adopts the perspective of individuals who are concerned about a loved one in the throes of depression. Dr. Noonan fluently guides the reader through a series of topics that, when taken together, provide a solid foundation for effectively supporting a loved one through a depressive illness.

Dr. Noonan begins by providing basic psychoeducation about mood disorders, including signs and symptoms to look for and how these may differ by age. From there, she describes skills to use when helping a loved one who is depressed, including: practicing active listening, setting boundaries, knowing when to consult professionals, responding effectively when someone refuses help, maintaining realistic expectations, fostering hope, and recognizing when the caregiver needs care. The final chapter, "Dos and Don'ts," is particularly appealing as a "cheat sheet."

In summary, this well-written and highly accessible volume provides essential background knowledge and a far-ranging but concise description of practical skills for those who love someone who is depressed. Dr. Noonan is a trustworthy guide, drawing from her experiences as physician, patient, caregiver, and speaker. She has created an insightful and compassionate manual for loved ones which we anticipate will be an encouraging and supportive resource for readers during an often challenging journey.

Timothy J. Petersen, PhD

Jonathan E. Alpert, MD, PhD

Andrew A. Nierenberg, MD

The Massachusetts General Hospital
Department of Psychiatry
Boston, Massachusetts

Preface

If you've chosen to open this book, you're in the company of many like you who are searching for ways to help a family member or a close friend who has depression or bipolar disorder. Perhaps in the past, you've felt awkward trying to help someone with such an emotionally charged problem. Maybe you weren't sure just what to say or do. Some people feel uncomfortable bringing up sensitive issues and can be at a loss for words in these situations. It's normal to worry about saying or doing the "wrong" thing and perhaps making the situation worse. This is a common fear.

You may have found that some circumstances require a delicate touch—one that you may not have a lot of experience with. In addition, if your family member is in a hot zone of emotion he may not be thinking clearly. He may misinterpret what you say or do. This can happen in the best of relationships.

Perhaps you've tried to talk to your friend or family member who is depressed and have felt shut out or excluded. Perhaps you're afraid that whatever you do isn't going to be helpful or make a difference, although you have good intentions. This can leave you feeling frustrated and powerless and eventually, worn out. When the problem is a mental illness, the stakes can be high. If someone close to you has depression or bipolar disorder, this book is for you. It will give you some ideas to help you know what to say and do.

Major depression and bipolar disorder are common biologically based conditions of the mind and body that affect the thoughts, feelings, actions, and everyday lives of many people. These two conditions, in a category called the *mood disorders*, are by nature often relapsing and remitting. This means that the symptoms can come and go over time in a pattern unique to each person. The fluctuations in your spouse or child or parent's illness may make it tough to predict what each day will be like. These mood changes can be very frustrating to watch, live with, and know how to handle.

While sitting in a roundtable discussion on mood disorders with parents, spouses, and patients at Massachusetts General Hospital in Boston, I heard serious frustration coming from the supporters of those who have depression and bipolar disorder. Family members and close friends are usually the first to recognize the symptoms of depression and the ones providing daily support. Most felt powerless to know what steps to take, what to say or do in response to symptoms, or how to change the course of the illness. I saw them struggle, too, with the unpredictable nature of mood disorders.

I know firsthand that many are looking for information on how to respond to the ups and downs of a loved one's mood disorder. Family members like you have few places to go for guidance on how to help. My goal in writing this book is to bring depression management strategies to those struggling to deal with this disabling illness in their spouse, sibling, parent, teenage or adult child, or close friend. In writing I draw on personal experience as a patient, provider, and caretaker; educational resources including evidence-based research; psychoeducational programs and seminars; experts in the field; and others' patient and family experiences. I offer recommendations on what to say and do when your family member or friend has depression-related difficulties. I also offer ways for you to foster resilience in those who have depression. I then focus on you, the caregiver or supporter, who personally feels the stress of the illness. You need assistance during these times and must learn to care for yourself as well.

This book is full of ideas for you to try. Some may work for you and your friend or family member; some may not. Not all families and relationships are alike or interact in the same way. You have to do what feels right for both of you. While there are similarities in how people experience depression, everyone is different. Each person also has her own way of communicating distress and accepting help. Some people are more private, some more talkative, and some more active. Attempt to understand your family member's unique style, reactions, and openness to receiving your help, and base your approach on that. Try something from this book that you think may be helpful, and see how she responds. Be careful not to force one idea on her, especially if it causes more agitation or withdrawal. If you find that one approach doesn't work, use another. Or change it slightly and try it another day. For example, if your spouse gets angry when you bring up his depression or if he considers it intrusive when you ask about his problems or how he is feeling, then stop and try a different approach. If he doesn't want to talk today, perhaps he'll go for a bike ride or a long walk with you. He may be ready to talk another day. Remember that you're there to support and love him—you don't have to try to be his therapist.

This book begins with an overview of major depression and bipolar disorder and gives you the background to better understand what you're dealing with. It also discusses the common symptoms of depression and the elevated mood of bipolar disorder using an easy-to-read table. The chapter also contains a section on the unique features of depression in adolescents, men, and women.

Chapter 2 explores Signs of Depression to Look For. This includes variations in your family member or friend's general appearance, vital senses (sleep habits, appetite), and attitude toward herself seen in depression. The second chapter also includes the Warning Signs of Suicide. It's helpful to become familiar with these Warning Signs so you know if it's ever time to take action.

Chapter 3 teaches the support skills and communication strategies uniquely helpful to caregivers of a person who has depression. It covers the skills of active listening and the empathic response. It offers concrete examples of what you might say and how you might handle certain situations.

Next, in chapter 4, you'll find Helpful Approaches that are useful in daily interactions with someone who has depression. These include treating him normally and not as a "sick" person, providing hope, having realistic expectations, confronting negative thoughts, knowing when to seek professional help, setting boundaries, and being familiar with the basic guidelines for promoting mental health.

Chapter 5 addresses the issue of Finding Professional Help. You'll learn how to determine when professional help is necessary. The chapter also shows how to choose a mental health provider who is a good fit for your family member and helps you realize what to expect afterward. It concludes with a section on When Someone Refuses Treatment, to help you understand the problem and know what steps to take.

Following that, chapter 6 presents What You Can Do Now to help your family member or friend. You'll learn to respond to any of the nine main symptoms of depression listed in the *Diagnostic and Statistical Manual of Mental Disorders* (*DSM-5*). It is the standard diagnostic manual in psychiatry.

Chapter 7, Anticipating Recovery—Skills to Have in Place, suggests how you can foster resilience in someone who has depression or bipolar disorder. *Resilience* is the skill of adapting well in the face of adversity and the ability to bounce back after difficult times, including an illness like a mood disorder. Depression is a relapsing and remitting illness that often challenges a person tremendously. Being able to weather its ups and downs will likely decrease the intensity of episodes and often improve your family member or friend's quality of life (Wingo et al. 2010).

Chapter 8 focuses on Caring for the Caregivers—you. It begins with a discussion on how depression in the family affects all members. Other topics include maintaining your own physical, emotional, and family health. This is essential to functioning well in a helper role.

Chapter 9 summarizes Dos and Don'ts, in a bulleted format for easy reference. I've also included a closing chapter to bring concepts together, a list of useful resources, and a glossary of terms.

One word of housekeeping. I understand that people reading this book are dealing with their spouse, significant other, adult or adolescent child, sister or brother, parent, aunt, uncle, grandparent, cousin, or close friend who has depression or bipolar disorder. The language can get rather cumbersome, and it's hard to choose one word that's all-inclusive to represent different family members. For this reason, throughout the book I vary the language, sometimes using a specific relationship and sometimes the grab-bag term "family member or friend." I also vary female and male pronouns, she and he. In almost all instances, I mean to include anyone who is affected by depression.

Acknowledgments

When I wrote my first book, *Managing Your Depression*, two years ago, I was stunned by the constellation of exceptional people who made it possible. I still am. They are all stars in my world. These professionals' superior clinical skills, kindness, understanding, and perseverance have continued to keep hope alive and growing for me when I believed there was none. I owe my deepest thanks and gratitude to Drs. Andrew Nierenberg, Jonathan Alpert, Timothy Petersen, and Karen Carlson. My family, father and brother, have been remarkably generous and supportive, and for that I am most grateful. And my friends, the ones who have sustained me throughout, deserve special thanks and appreciation: Sandi, Ginger, Cindy, Dave, Carol, Marty, JoAnn, Joe, and Dan D.

The insightful Jacqueline Wehmueller and staff of Johns Hopkins University Press also deserve special recognition. They took me through the amazing journey of my first, and now second, book with perceptive and thoughtful care. No book is published alone.

When Someone You Know Has Depression

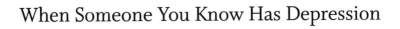

Introduction

Mood disorders are considered among the most disabling of all medical conditions. A leading cause of suicide, they have an impact on nearly every level of an affected person's functioning. Depression affects about 350 million people of all ages worldwide (World Health Organization 2015). An estimated 16 million adults and 2.2 million adolescents experienced at least one major depressive episode in the United States in 2012 (National Institute of Mental Health 2015). Bipolar disorder (bipolar I, II, and bipolar spectrum) affects another 4.5 percent of adults.

These large numbers may be surprising. People often hide their illness and do not speak openly of it for a variety of reasons. The fear of being stigmatized—of being unfairly labeled or stereotyped—is the most common. Stigma, or unfounded judgment and criticism based on misinformation, upsets the lives of many people with mental illness and causes great anxiety. Even though we've made great strides in understanding mood disorders as a medical condition, those affected still face discrimination both socially and in the workplace.

Mental health researchers commonly report that women experience symptoms of depression twice as often as men. In 2012 in the United States, 8.4 percent of adult women and 5.2 percent of adult men had at least one major depressive episode (National Institute of Mental Health 2015). At the same time, 13.7 percent of adolescent girls and 4.7 percent of adolescent boys had at least one major depressive episode (National Institute of Mental Health 2015). These differences may be related to issues common to women, including the stress of family and social obligations and hormone fluctuations during the menstrual cycle, before and after childbirth (as in postpartum depression), and during menopause.

However, some in psychiatry wonder if these numbers are accurate. They question whether or not we are identifying all of the instances of depression in men. For example, it might just *look* as if women experience twice the rate of depression as men. This is because men may experience different symptoms or fail to report the traditional symptoms of depression, such as sadness, fatigue, loss of interest, sleep, or appetite. Most men find admitting to sadness or crying socially unacceptable. They are often brought up to withhold their feelings. Men who experience emotional distress may also be more likely to react with anger, aggression, irritability, or self-destructive and risk-taking behavior. They may numb their pain with alcohol, drugs, gambling, or excess work.

In 2013 University of Michigan researchers looked at whether men and women experience depression equally (Martin, Neighbors, and Griffith 2013). They gathered information using a self-report questionnaire of English-speaking adults in the United States. First, they looked at gender differences in depression symptoms using a rating scale. They found that "male specific" symptoms such as anger, aggression, alcohol and substance use, irritability, and risk-taking behavior were more common in men than women.

The researchers then combined these symptoms with fifteen traditional symptoms of depression in a new rating scale. Men and women met the definition for depression in fairly equal numbers when measured using this combined rating scale. The researchers believe that current depression screening, which relies only on traditional symptoms, may fail to include symptoms common to men. As a result, depression in men may be underreported. More studies are needed to fully understand which symptoms accurately identify depression in men and to learn if men and women experience depression in equal proportions.

There are some limitations to this study. It is a "secondary data analysis" study, which means that it was planned out in advance and information was collected and analyzed after the fact. The authors were able to evaluate most but not all potential symptoms of depression. Also, there were two time frames for answering the study questions ("in your lifetime" and "in the past thirty days"). None of this affects the point of the study for our purpose.

In keeping with the numbers showing women's higher depression rates, three times more women than men attempt suicide. However, four times as many men die by suicide. In 2013, there were 41,149 persons who committed suicide in the United States (American Foundation for Suicide Prevention 2015, data from the Centers for Disease Control and Prevention). Of those, 77.9 percent were male and 22.1 percent were female. Firearms were the most common method (51.4 percent), followed by suffocation (24.5 percent) and poisoning (16.1 percent).

No accurate numbers exist for those who have tried to seriously harm themselves or attempt suicide. The Centers for Disease Control and Prevention gathers information from hospitals on nonfatal injuries that occur from self-harm. In 2013, there were 494,169 visits to a hospital in the United States for injuries due to self-harm (American Foundation for Suicide Prevention 2015). While many suicide attempts go unreported or untreated, surveys suggest that at least 1 million people harm themselves each year in the United States, at a medical cost of $2 billion per year (American Foundation for Suicide Prevention 2015).

Most people with depression don't experience this illness alone. They have family members and close friends, like you, who care and want to know what they can do to help. In fact, depression and bipolar disorder are considered family illnesses, for two main reasons. First, depression can be genetic, or run in families. Second, it usually affects a person's friends or family in some negative way. You and other family members may feel emotionally down, put off, shut out, worn out, or guilty from dealing with a mood disorder in your loved one twenty-four hours a day. You may feel you've done something to cause her unhappiness, isolation, or irritability. You may find that your family plans are frequently interrupted, personal finances are affected, and more of your energy goes toward dealing with her life issues. There may be more stress in the family in having to cope with a member who is ill. The family may experience added burdens as health insurers and HMOs fail to fully understand the person's medical needs and the level of care required.

It is not easy to help someone with any medical problem, including a mental health disorder like depression and bipolar disorder. It's difficult for caregivers in your position to find the balance between providing much-needed help to a family member and supporting her sense of independence. You may feel burned out from the work and effort if the illness lasts for a long time. Most important, helping someone who has a mood disorder is and feels different from caring for a person with other medical problems. It carries with it special challenges:

Turning down help. With depression, it may not be as simple as asking your family member or friend "How can I help?" and receiving feedback on what you can do. You may instead hear, "Leave me alone," "I just want to stay in bed," "You don't understand," or "There's nothing anyone can do to help." Unlike other illnesses, someone who has depression may reject help rather than welcome it. This is because depression affects a person's mind and thinking.

Your friend or family member may be unable to cope using her regular methods of dealing with other illness or stress. She may feel far beyond any hope or help. She might believe that even if she were to get better, she has nothing to offer anyone and will never have a life worth living, a meaningful career, or a fulfilling relationship. She could feel fundamentally flawed and defective, unlovable, and incompetent. Or she may be convinced that this is a permanent state that will never improve. Even if she has successfully overcome depression before, it's not uncommon for her to forget ever having felt well and deny it.

In depression, it's hard for the affected person to separate the illness symptoms from "just me." She may believe that her current state is her normal, usual self and forget what she was like before the depression episode. For example, she may not recall that she ever had a sense of humor or was good at making friends. If your family member has bipolar disorder and is in a manic state, she may also lose *insight*, that special sense of self-awareness and perspective, and deny that she has an illness at all. She may angrily reject help, believing you're the one with the problem, misguided and narrow minded. This makes your job all the more difficult.

Stigma and misunderstanding. Symptoms of depression often overlap with normal feelings such as sadness or fatigue, making it difficult to know what's really going on. We now know that depression is a biologic medical condition. Even so, it's not unusual for people to wonder whether their family member or friend who has depression really has an illness. They may believe he is just lazy or lacks ambition. You might sometimes feel that your family member or friend is simply not trying hard enough to get better. Perhaps you think he could just "snap out of it" if he really wanted to. This can happen even if you are knowledgeable about depression and have only the best intentions.

I encourage you to let go of your guilt about having these thoughts on occasion, especially in private moments when you are tired and stressed. It's easy to understand depression as an illness when you're distanced from it. It is much more difficult to keep that in mind when you're living with someone day to day who has depression. Just try to be aware of these thoughts, and recognize that such thoughts are not helpful and only contribute to the stress of caring for your family member.

Be aware, too, that mistaken beliefs about depression often complicate its treatment. Most of us would encourage someone to take prescribed medications for diabetes, high blood pressure, or bronchitis. However, it's not uncommon for us to question whether treatments for depression are necessary, whether they are a crutch or a Band-Aid or perhaps even addictive. Even if you realize the errors in these statements, you know that others may wonder whether your family member "really needs to be taking those drugs." They may even urge him to stop taking them, against all medical advice. Gaining the support of these family members and friends can be difficult. This makes it harder for you and your family member to stick with the recommended treatment.

Confidentiality and sharing information. Current federal regulations address the privacy of health information. These regulations are stricter for mental health disorders than for other medical conditions. This means that your family member's doctors or counselors are not allowed to share information with you without her explicit permission. This applies even if she is hospitalized in a psychiatric unit. As a result, you may feel shut out from her evaluation and treatment. You may also wonder whether the treatment team thinks you caused or contributed to your family member's depression. However, in an emergency you can speak with her doctors. You can contribute valuable information about her, particularly when she can't communicate clearly herself. The treatment provider can receive this information without violating her privacy concerns. Mental health professionals will welcome your support and the perspective you provide as an ally in treatment.

Uncertain outcome. Although the treatment and outcome for medical problems such as a knee replacement or strep throat varies, there are still reliable guidelines and expectations for these conditions. Doctors can usually provide helpful guidance about the recovery time in days, weeks, or months. If you are helping a family member through one of these conditions, you can usually plan your life around it. However, this is much more difficult to do with depression or bipolar disorder. Some people respond to the first treatment and are back to their old selves in a few months. Others don't respond as readily and have a more complicated treatment course. They may need to try many different medications and treatments. Their diagnosis may need refining over time, as more information becomes available. This can become a long, unpredictable journey. It's wise to attend to your own health and well-being in order to be able to support your family member during his recovery.

Lack of established routines. We usually know how to respond when a friend or family member has a serious medical problem like cancer, a heart attack, or other medical problem. We organize rides to appointments, accompany her to chemotherapy, and sit with her for hours as she recovers from its side effects. We bring casseroles and funny movies and organize fundraising walks. We know when to call 9-1-1. In contrast, we're not yet comfortable in knowing just what to do for a person with depression or bipolar disorder. I wrote this book because I realized how you, as a well-meaning friend or family member, can spring into action when you are familiar with the diagnosis and how to help, but often withdraw and don't know just what to do when it's a mood disorder.

Now that we've looked at who gets depression and bipolar disorder and how they affect the person and his family and friends, it's time to look at what we can do and say, as family members and friends, to help the person get better. We begin with the symptoms of depression and how they vary among people.

CHAPTER 1

What Are Mood Disorders?

We'll begin our journey with a review of mood disorders. Having background information about depression and bipolar disorder will help you better understand the condition. You'll have an idea of what your family member or friend is experiencing and feeling. That understanding, in turn, will help you say and do what will be most helpful. Many people like you have found this to be true.

As mentioned earlier, *mood disorders* are a category of psychiatric conditions that include both major depression and bipolar disorder. Mood disorders involve our state of mind—the part of our inner self that colors and drives our thoughts, feelings, and behaviors. They are biologically based, treatable illnesses that affect all aspects of our lives.

Normally, our mood changes over time and across a broad range of emotions. It can be described using any number of words: up, down, neutral, happy, sad, and others. When we're depressed, our mood is persistently very down, and our mental and physical functioning is not as sharp as usual. We don't think as clearly, organize ourselves, or do things as well as before. A negative mood may be related to *external* or *internal* events in our lives. External events are things that happen to us. A job loss, a relationship break-up, or a visit with a controlling parent are examples of negative external events. Internal events include thoughts and feelings inside us, like believing we are unlovable or undesirable.

External and internal events can act as triggers to cause a change in our mood. *Triggers* are events or circumstances that may cause a person distress and increase his depression symptoms. Common triggers include stressful life events both positive (a birth or moving to a new home) and negative (a death or divorce), conflicts, inter-personal stress, changes in sleep, or substance abuse. Sometimes we cannot identify the trigger that happens before an episode of depression. A dark mood may come on gradually, or it may feel rather sudden after a period of subtle life events.

Each person has his own set of unique triggers. It is helpful for you to become familiar with those events that cause your family member distress. When you see a trigger affecting him or coming up in the future, try to make sure he is receiving treatment, taking his medications, managing life's stressors, seeing his mental health professional, and following the Basics of Mental Health (discussed in chapter 4).

Depression and Bipolar Disorder

Major Depression

Major depression is also called *depression, major depressive disorder,* or *unipolar depression.* The symptoms of major depression are broad; they negatively affect your family member or friend's thoughts, feelings, behaviors, physical self, interests, activities, and relationships. A person with depression often has difficulty with basic everyday functioning, doing things for himself, or concentrating and making decisions. These are symptoms of the illness and are not signs of laziness. They are not intentional.

You may be familiar with the image of a depressed person feeling sad and losing interest in activities. We all feel a little sad at times, but that sadness is different; it is not depression. Rather, depression is a biologically based medical condition whose symptoms run deeper and last longer than you might expect. Your family member or friend may not feel well or like himself at the start of his illness but may be able to carry on with his usual daily activities. For example, he may wake up and get dressed and go through the motions of his day, without much interest or energy. He may feel it's a bit of a struggle to accomplish all the tasks he used to do; the flavor for life has left him. He might not fully understand what is happening to him. The person who has depression is often the last one to realize what is going on. He may deny that he's even experiencing depression.

The American Psychiatric Association's (APA) *Diagnostic and Statistical Manual of Mental Disorders* (*DSM-5*) describes depression. It states that a person must have at least five of the following nine symptoms, lasting 2 weeks or longer (at least one of the five symptoms must be either persistent sadness or loss of interest), to be diagnosed with depression:

- Persistent sadness, hopelessness, and irritability
- Loss of enjoyment and interest in activities that used to be pleasurable
- Loss of appetite or increased appetite, unintentional weight loss due to lack of interest in food, or weight gain
- Trouble falling asleep or staying asleep, light sleep, sleeping too much or too little, or waking up earlier than necessary
- Feelings of physical agitation or restlessness or of being physically slowed down
- Fatigue or loss of energy for no reason
- Feelings of worthlessness or guilt without foundation
- Decreased ability to focus and concentrate, or read
- Recurrent thoughts of death or suicide with or without a plan, or a suicide attempt

Depression Symptoms Can Vary

Depression is most often a *relapsing* and *remitting* illness. This means that it can come and go over time. That is often very frustrating for you and your family member or friend. Depression symptoms come in episodes that may last from several weeks to several months or longer. Each episode can vary in the length of time it lasts and how deep (or severe) it is. The intervals between episodes of depression also vary. Many people have repeat episodes of depression and may feel and function well in between. Others have a few residual symptoms in the intervals between episodes. The pattern of episodes is unique to each person.

You can better understand your family member or friend's pattern of depression by having him record his moods each day on a Mood Chart (see pages 16 and 17). This may help him connect his depression symptoms to life events or changes in medications. It is also a good way to follow his progress and response to treatment. Sharing this information with his treatment providers can help them make sound treatment decisions. It can also provide a basis of discussion in therapy sessions.

Relapse and Recurrence

As noted above, depression and bipolar disorder are not always one-time experiences. Not what you wanted to hear, I know. Even those who are successfully treated and recover from an episode many have a repeat episode, called a *relapse* or *recurrence*. A relapse is the return of full depressive symptoms after *partial recovery* from an episode. A recurrence is the return of full depressive symptoms following a *full recovery* from an episode.

Sixty percent of those who have had one episode of depression and recover will have a second at some time in their life. Seventy percent of those with two episodes will experience a third, and 90 percent of those with three episodes will have a fourth (Yeung, Feldman, and Fava 2010). Don't be disheartened. Depression is treatable and the symptoms can be managed. *Cognitive Behavioral Therapy* (CBT), a type of talk therapy that addresses the connection between our thoughts, feelings, and behaviors, and *Mindfulness-based CBT* can decrease the chance of relapse and recurrence (Fava et al. 1998; Teasdale et al. 2000).

Treatment-Resistant Depression

You may have heard the common complaint "Antidepressants don't work." You may have also seen the term *treatment-resistant depression*. This implies that, despite trying various medications and treatments, the person has not seen improvement in his depression symptoms or level of functioning. Until recently it was thought that many people who have difficult-to-treat or treatment-resistant depression are inadequately treated or undertreated. It might be that someone's medication dosage is too low. Or he just hasn't been on it long enough to give it a chance to work. He may not tolerate it very well and stop taking it early because of side effects. Perhaps it's not the best choice of drug for his particular symptoms. Now, new medications that are better tolerated, combined with careful attention to treatment guidelines by providers, have changed this thinking.

Currently, psychiatrists see many people who fail to respond or achieve remission after an adequate course of treatment. *Response* is defined as a partial improvement in symptoms; *remission* is complete relief, free of depression symptoms (Nierenberg and De-Cecco 2001). There is no single definition of or accepted diagnostic criteria for treatment-resistant depression. It may mean failure to improve after one course of an antidepressant of adequate dose and duration, or it may mean failure to respond to three or more courses of antidepressants and other treatments, including talk therapy or electroconvulsive therapy (ECT) over several months or more.

The reality is that only 50 percent of those who have depression respond to a first course of antidepressant treatment, and only 33 percent achieve full remission after a first course (Trivedi et al. 2006). Response to treatment often takes weeks or months. For many, it takes multiple attempts at treatment to reach a satisfactory response or recovery. This can all be discouraging for you and your family member. Choosing a treatment plan for depression is complex and takes great effort, even for trained psychiatrists. A consultation with an experienced psychiatrist to review medications and other treatment can be quite valuable.

Medication options for treatment-resistant depression can be to (1) switch to another antidepressant, (2) augment the antidepressant drug by adding a non-antidepressant drug to enhance the effects of the antidepressant drug, or (3) combine different types of antidepressants. Other treatment options might include psychotherapy or neurostimulation, a method that uses low electrical or magnetic current to stimulate the mood centers of the brain. These can be either non-invasive or invasive therapies. Non-invasive examples include electroconvulsive therapy and repetitive transcranial magnetic stimulation (rTMS). Invasive therapies such as deep brain stimulation require brain surgery and are not considered lightly. Chapter 5 has more information about these therapies. Even when they are under the care of experts, some individuals may be difficult to treat—may be considered to be treatment resistant. Psychiatrists urge the person who has depression not to despair or give up on treatment.

How to Use the Mood Chart

Encourage your family member or friend to use the Mood Chart every day for a month. It's easy. All he needs to do is check the box that best describes his mood that day. For example, he might choose a depressed mood that he estimates to be *severe, moderate,* or *mild*. Have him make the best guess. It doesn't have to be exact. A sample completed Mood Chart is provided on page 16.

The Mood Chart may help your family member or friend track fluctuations in his illness and identify patterns in his mood over a month's time. It is a better reflection of his illness than trying to remember these details during a doctor's appointment. The "Notes" column on the Mood Chart is meant to record anything that may have affected his mood that day, such as a change in medications or a stressful event. Women might record hormonal changes or a menstrual period. A blank Mood Chart is provided on page 17.

As you can see after filling in the Mood Chart, the course of depression typically has ups and downs. In addition, each of your family member or friend's symptoms can separately vary in how deep or severe it feels. This means he could experience a range of feelings or behaviors for each particular symptom.

For example, if he has a "depressed mood or irritability," he could feel anywhere from slightly blue to overwhelmingly down, devastated and unable to function, or somewhere in between. Many people find this kind of variation to be true. Or he could either have a slight to moderate "loss of appetite" or perhaps lose 10 pounds over 2 weeks because he lacks all interest in food. Table 1.1 gives examples of the variations you might see within each symptom of depression.

Why is this important? The variations in symptoms and their pattern are unique to every person and are unpredictable. Your friend or family member's doctors will be helped greatly in deciding on the best course of treatment if they can see his symptom variations.

The Theory of Depression

Imagine the brain as a network of brain cells (called *neurons*) bathed in special chemicals that help the cells communicate with each other. One long-held view is that depression disrupts these chemicals, called *neurotransmitters*, found in the part of the brain that regulates emotions and behavior. The chemical disruption is thought to happen when certain life events occur in a susceptible person.

A more recent theory of depression involves the interaction of our genes and the events in our life (Saveanu and Nemeroff 2012). A *gene* is a precise arrangement of molecules (a sequence of DNA) that make up the chromosomes in our cells. Genes instruct the body to make certain proteins to control our normal bodily functions, including our brain. Genes are inherited from our parents. Scientists have now found genes associated with particular diseases, such as Huntington's Disease, cystic fibrosis, and others. Some genes are believed to be associated with psychiatric illnesses such as schizophrenia, bipolar disorder, and depression. Eleven genes associated with susceptibility to bipolar disorder have been found. Identifying this information and understanding how it affects us may help in designing new interventions and treatments.

Sample Completed Mood Chart

Day	Depressed			Neutral	Elevated Mood			Notes
	severe	moderate	mild	neutral	mild	moderate	severe	
1	√							
2	√							
3		√						Argument with father
4		√						
5		√						
6		√						
7	√							
8	√							
9	√							Added new medication
10		√						
11		√						
12		√						
13			√					
14			√					
15			√					
16		√						
17			√					
18			√					
19				√				
20				√				
21			√					
22								
23								
24								
25								
26								
27								
28								
29								
30								
31								

Source: Susan J. Noonan, *Managing Your Depression: What You Can Do to Feel Better* (Johns Hopkins University Press, 2013), 46.

Blank Mood Chart

Day	Depressed			Neutral	Elevated Mood			Notes
	severe	moderate	mild	neutral	mild	moderate	severe	
1								
2								
3								
4								
5								
6								
7								
8								
9								
10								
11								
12								
13								
14								
15								
16								
17								
18								
19								
20								
21								
22								
23								
24								
25								
26								
27								
28								
29								
30								
31								

Source: Susan J. Noonan, *Managing Your Depression: What You Can Do to Feel Better* (Johns Hopkins University Press, 2013), 46.

Table 1.1. Intensity of Depression Symptoms

Symptoms of depression	Family member isn't bothered too much by depression and he ...	Family member is affected by depression in many areas of his life and he ...	Family member is very much affected by depression and he ...
Depressed mood, hopelessness, or irritability	Is dispirited but still functioning	Feels sad and unhappy most of time or irritable	Looks and feels totally miserable; unable to function
Diminished interest or pleasure in things	Has reduced interest in things	Has greater loss of interest or pleasure	Is unable to feel any emotion or pleasure
Weight loss or gain OR increased or decreased appetite	Has mild loss of taste	Lost or gained 2–5 lbs. unintentionally; no appetite	Lost or gained 5 lb. or more unintentionally; needs persuasion to eat
Sleeping too much OR too little	Has slight difficulty falling asleep or sleeps lightly	Has several awakenings interrupting sleep (~ 2 hours)	Sleeps 2–3 hours per night OR over 10 hours total
Physical restlessness OR slowing down	Has difficulty starting activities	Finds activities are carried out with great effort	Is unable to do anything without help OR is pacing, restless
Fatigue or loss of energy nearly every day	Has difficulty starting activities	Finds activities are carried out with great effort	Is unable to do anything without help
Feelings of worthlessness or guilt	Occasionally feels worthless	Frequently feels worthless or guilty	Has frequent and intrusive thoughts of worthlessness
Diminished ability to think or concentrate; make decisions	Has occasional and mild episodes	Has frequent and marked episodes	Has this every day and it's intrusive; is unable to read or converse normally
Recurrent thoughts of death or suicide, a plan, or a suicide attempt	Has fleeting thoughts of suicide	Has common thoughts but no specific suicide plans or intention	Has explicit plans for suicide

Environmental events are the things, people, and life events that go on around us, both inside and outside our bodies. The *gene x environment* theory of depression is thought to work as follows: Our genes interact with our environment and life experiences to shape the network of cells in our brain. The shaping is thought to occur because the brain is sensitive to stress and traumatic events during vulnerable periods of our life. Stress or illness cause negative stimulation and can activate certain genes or change the action of genes. This is important because these are the genes that affect the normal functioning of our brain. If stress or illness changes gene activity during a vulnerable period, the genes and brain do not work as well. Depression can result. Depression is not entirely genetic and is not entirely related to life experiences. It requires both at a time when the person is vulnerable.

Depression is also thought to run in some families. A person can inherit genetic factors that make him more likely to experience depression. But this does not guarantee he will have the illness. He may not have an episode of depression unless he experiences certain stressful life events during a vulnerable period in his life, when the genes affect brain functioning. Some examples of stressful life events include major emotional trauma (a major loss or the death of a loved one), chronic stress, hormonal changes, physical illness, sleep disorders, substance abuse, and others.

What does it feel like for your family member who has depression? Depression is not just "feeling blue" or mopey for a day or two. It is different from grief, which has a focus, a beginning and an end. Rather, for many people depression is a period of deep despair. They see no end in sight, no hope for their future, and no possibility of relief from their fatigue and suffering. They often feel both physical and emotional pain and cannot participate in life. A person who has depression sees only the dark, negative side of the world. He experiences life in a distorted way, with a negative view of himself, his future, and the world. At times he may feel irritable and take it out on those around him, starting arguments about little things. This is not intentional. He may withdraw from life, friends, and activities. He may lose friends. Communication is often a major effort when depressed.

Your family member may lose interest in the things around him, stop enjoying his past interests, and feel little motivation to participate in life. Sleep and appetite may be markedly affected. He may not sleep except in short naps, or he may sleep too much. Food may be tasteless, or he may binge on junk food as an easy way to ease his pain. Fatigue frequently sets in and compounds the mood symptoms.

Focus and concentration are a challenge to many people with depression, and his thinking may slow down or become disorganized. This can make work and school difficult and frustrating, particularly for someone used to functioning at a high level. Projects and work often pile up, the mail remains unopened, and the household chores get neglected. He may spend hours just staring straight ahead, unable to tackle the task before him. Some people think about death to relieve their emotional pain. Table 1.2 will give you an idea of the type of depression symptoms your family member or friend may have. It shows you the range of thoughts, feelings, and behaviors that characterize this illness.

Depression can be very rough on a family, especially the primary support person. The fluctuating moods of your family member who has depression may add to the stress of a busy household. This can affect everyone around him. It requires time and patience on your part to understand what is going on at the moment, know whether something has triggered an episode, and decide how best to respond. You may have many emotions yourself, such as frustration, anger, or guilt. You must be careful to attend to your own and other family members' needs as well and avoid burnout. For more on this topic refer to chapter 8, Caring for the Caregivers.

Bipolar Disorder

Bipolar disorder, known as *manic depressive disorder* in the past, is another mood disorder. Like depression, it is a relapsing and

Table 1.2. Symptoms of Depression

Negative thoughts

__ I deserve this.	__ I'm not as good as everyone else.
__ I'm being punished.	__ Nobody will ever care about me.
__ It's all my fault.	__ I'm worthless.
__ I can't make decisions.	__ People are against me.
__ I can't remember anything.	__ I should be _____ by now.
__ Nothing good will ever happen.	__ I've wasted my (life, education, opportunities).
__ Things will never get better.	__ There is no hope for me.
__ I never do anything right.	__ I think about dying or suicide a lot.

Feelings

__ I feel sad for no reason.	__ I feel easily annoyed or irritated.
__ I don't feel good even if good things happen.	__ I fear that something terrible will happen.
__ I feel worthless.	__ I feel tired all the time.
__ I feel bad; inferior to other people.	__ I'm not interested in anything.
__ I feel guilty about everything.	__ I'm not interested in sex.

Behaviors

__ I cry a lot for no reason.	__ I've stopped my previous activities and hobbies.
__ I sleep too much.	__ I've stopped exercising.
__ I sleep too little.	__ I argue and fight with people for no reason.
__ I eat too much.	__ I'm fidgety and restless.
__ I eat very little.	__ I move or speak slowly.
__ I drink too much alcohol.	__ I have trouble concentrating.
__ I've recently gained a lot of weight.	__ I have difficulty reading the newspaper or following shows on television.
__ I recently lost a lot of weight without trying.	__ I can't keep track of my thoughts to have a conversation.
__ I stay in bed or on the couch all day.	__ My house is more disorganized than usual.
__ Sometimes I don't take a shower, wash my hair, or shave.	__ I forget to pay bills.
__ I have trouble starting or finishing projects.	__ I forget to do or don't do laundry or other household duties.
__ I avoid people and isolate myself.	__ I call in sick to work or school a lot.
__ I don't return telephone calls.	

Source: Susan J. Noonan, *Managing Your Depression: What You Can Do to Feel Better* (Johns Hopkins University Press, 2013), 43.

remitting illness with a significant impact on daily life. Bipolar disorder is thought to be associated with genes that interfere with the normal functioning of the brain. It is characterized by periodic episodes of extreme elevated mood or irritability, called *manic episodes*, followed by episodes of extreme depression, or *bipolar depression*. These episodes come in cycles; the pattern differs for each person. The symptoms of bipolar depression are very similar to those of major depression. It takes time and the skills of an experienced mental health professional to make an accurate diagnosis between the two. Moreover, the treatment for each is very different.

The *DSM-5* states that to be diagnosed with a bipolar manic episode, a person must experience an elevated or irritable mood that impairs functioning and lasts for at least 1 week, as well as at least three of the following symptoms:

- Inflated sense of self or grandiosity
- Increased physical and mental activity and agitated body movements (*psychomotor agitation*)
- Decreased need for sleep
- Racing thoughts
- Easily distracted with poor concentration
- Pressured speech, which is a certain way of being more talkative than usual (rapid, loud, nonstop talking)
- Irritability
- High-risk behaviors (excessive spending, impulsive sexual behavior, etc.)

The different types of bipolar disorder, called *bipolar I*, *bipolar II*, *bipolar spectrum*, and *mixed states*, cross a spectrum of these symptoms. The bipolar type depends on the depth and length of time the elevated mood symptoms last. A person who has bipolar I typically has manic episodes and depressive episodes. People who have bipolar II have hypomanic episodes and prolonged depressive episodes. The symptoms of bipolar spectrum fall somewhere in between. A *manic episode* is as described above. A *hypomanic episode* is less intense and shorter in length, and *mixed states* are a combination of mania (or hypomania) and depression at the same time. Table 1.3 provides examples of the symptoms of an elevated mood.

What does it feel like for your family member or friend who has bipolar disorder? Most find it very difficult to go through the different phases of mania, hypomania, depression, or a mixed state. Bipolar depression is very similar to major depression. During this time he may withdraw from friends and family. He may feel too irritable to be around people. Problems with concentration and focus can affect his work or school. Symptoms of fatigue, sadness, loss of interest, loss of appetite, and sleep disturbances are common. Negative thinking dominates in many people during the depressed phase.

At the other extreme, a manic or hypomanic episode is often described as having a storm inside one's head. Characteristically, when a person is manic, his thoughts and speech race from idea to idea without completing a thought. Your family member or friend might be too disorganized and distracted to function well but fails to realize it. In fact, like many in the manic phase, he may believe he can do anything—and do it extraordinarily well. This is not actually the case.

Your family member or friend may feel energized, with little or no need for sleep. He might engage in impulsive, high-risk behaviors, such as compulsive shopping and spending money, excessive drinking, illegal drug use, reckless driving, or extreme sexual behavior. His actions could potentially lead to poor social, financial, and business decisions. They affect the person with bipolar disorder and everyone around him.

Depression in Men

Some men who have depression exhibit irritability and agitation, rather than sadness, as their major symptom of a mood disorder. Your family member may appear cranky and irritable instead of sad or tearful when depressed. Irritability can lead him to persistently direct angry outbursts or frustration over minor matters toward

Table 1.3. Symptoms of Elevated Mood

Elevated thoughts	
__ I have special abilities. __ I have a lot of good ideas. __ My thoughts are really great. __ Many people are interested in me and my ideas. __ Many people are against me. __ I get very focused on a project or cause.	__ My thoughts jump around quickly from one topic to another. __ Other people say they can't follow what I'm saying. __ The rest of the world is too slow. __ It takes others a really long time to do things.

Feelings	
__ I feel good even when bad things happen. __ I feel happy without reason. __ I'm very self-confident. __ I feel like I have lots of energy even when I get less sleep than usual. __ I feel optimistic about everything.	__ I feel great, on top of the world. __ I feel that everything will go my way. __ I feel that nothing bad can happen to me. __ I feel that I'm easily annoyed or irritated. __ I'm very impatient. __ I feel more interested in sex than usual.

Behaviors	
__ I sleep less than usual but don't feel tired. __ I laugh a lot or for no reason. __ I'm more talkative than usual. __ I'm fidgety, restless, and I pace. __ I have trouble concentrating. __ I'm easily distracted. __ I start lots of new projects and activities. __ I've increased my activities, work, and hobbies. __ I don't finish projects before starting new ones. __ I'm much more sociable than usual. __ I make more phone calls than usual.	__ I spend money and go on shopping sprees. __ I make impulsive decisions. __ I tip excessively and gamble. __ I take more risks than usual. __ I do more risky or dangerous activities. __ I start arguments or fights for no reason. __ I drive fast. __ I've increased my use of alcohol or drugs. __ I dress flashier than usual. __ My handwriting has gotten larger and messier.

Source: Susan J. Noonan, *Managing Your Depression: What You Can Do to Feel Better* (Johns Hopkins University Press, 2013), 44.

others. Sometimes, he won't be able to tolerate another person nearby, even if he knows you mean well.

Men often have more anger attacks, acts of aggression, substance abuse issues, and risk-taking behaviors than women (Martin, Neighbors, and Griffith 2013). Some may scream and yell; argue; break things; engage in risky behaviors such as gambling, drinking, or substance abuse; engage in excessive sexual behavior; or work too much as a sign of depression. An agitated depression can be very difficult to treat because your family member or friend's actions can be unpredictable.

Depression in Adolescents

Irritability and agitation may also be the primary feature in your child or adolescent. You may notice a difference in his school or work performance, a loss of friends or a new crowd of friends, or a change in activities he once enjoyed. Your teenager might be more withdrawn and secretive about what he does and where he goes—and with whom. He may become argumentative and fight with you or his siblings.

Your daughter may become tearful and withdrawn, especially around the time of menstruation. Some adolescents may miss days of school or work or take a temporary leave of absence from school. Alcohol, illegal drugs, and reckless driving can become issues. The important thing is that you notice and respond to any unusual changes in your adolescent's typical emotion and behavior.

Depression in Women

Some women find that their mood symptoms change as *estrogen* and *progesterone*, the reproductive hormones produced in the ovaries, shift throughout their life (Sichel and Driscoll 1999). This may happen right before their menstrual period, when it is called *premenstrual syndrome*, or PMS. PMS refers to a pattern of physical, emotional, and behavioral symptoms that occur 1 to 2 weeks before the menstrual period and end when the period begins. Symptoms include anger, anxiety, depression, irritability, poor concentration, bloating, breast tenderness, fatigue, and muscle aches. *Premenstrual dysphoric disorder* (PMDD) is a more severe form of PMS, with irritability as its hallmark symptom. Women may also experience depression during pregnancy or after childbirth, when it's known as *postpartum depression*. It is related to a rapid shift in hormones a woman is experiencing. Symptoms may be mild, with bouts of tearfulness, or deep and extreme.

If the woman who has depression is a wife, mother, or pregnant, her illness can affect the entire family. Children growing up in a household where the mother has depression or bipolar disorder may experience a variety of emotional problems themselves (Barker et al. 2012; Batten et al. 2012; Pilowsky et al. 2006; Weissman et al. 2004). A spouse or significant other can also feel the effects.

Some women going through *menopause* may have episodes of depression. During menopause, the body naturally slows its reproductive hormone cycles, and a woman stops having menstrual periods. Depression at this time is called *peri-menopausal*, *menopausal*, or *postmenopausal* depression. Menopause begins, on average, at age 47 and lasts 4 to 8 years. Peri-menopause begins 3 to 5 years before menopause, when estrogen levels begin to slowly drop. Postmenopause occurs when a woman's monthly periods finally stop. Some women experience depression during these times.

The decline in the function of the ovaries causes them to make less estrogen (or *estradiol*). This may trigger depression in some vulnerable women (Schmidt et al. 2015). Symptoms can include fatigue, trouble sleeping, difficulty with concentration and remembering small details, hot flashes, night sweats, and mood shifts. Episodes of depression can be less frequent and may sometimes disappear once a woman passes through menopause.

The exact relationship between mood and hormones is not fully understood, but research is ongoing. The Massachusetts General Hospital Center for Women's Mental Health Web site at www.womensmentalhealth.org is a valuable resource on women and depression. Here, you will find a library of information, a newsletter, and a blog covering up-to-date topics, including depression and

PMS and PMDD, peri-natal and postpartum depression, fertility and mental health, and menopausal symptoms.

Symptoms of Advanced Depression

There are some rare times when a person who has depression or bipolar disorder may have such distorted thoughts that he loses touch with reality. His perception of the world becomes wildly inaccurate. These are called *psychotic features* and indicate severe illness. For example, he may see or hear things that are not actually there, called *hallucinations*. They are very real to him, and the concern is that he could act upon what he believes he is "told" to do.

He may have paranoid delusions and believe he is being stalked or followed, that the FBI is tapping his telephone, or that his body organs are decaying inside him. In the mania of bipolar disorder, he might be convinced that he has superhuman powers and can do anything extraordinarily well. Any of these features constitute a psychiatric emergency. The person needs immediate evaluation and treatment by a mental health professional.

Anxiety and Depression

Approximately half those people who have depression experience anxiety at the same time (Regier et al. 1998). *Anxiety* is a feeling of excessive nervousness, apprehension, and worry about the future. The depth of worry, length of time it lasts, and how often it occurs is out of proportion to the actual feared event. It may cause your family member or friend a great deal of distress. Worry leads to a nervous and jittery feeling. He may feel restless and shaky, with trouble concentrating, irritability, and sleep difficulties. Physically, your family member could feel sweaty, shaky, and like his heart is racing or skipping a beat. An upset stomach, nausea, headache, and muscle aches are common. It all feels very real to the person at the time. Some people are frightened by these symptoms and go to the Emergency Department thinking that something is wrong with them physically.

Anxiety is a treatable condition. Medications, talk therapy, relaxation exercises, and mindfulness meditation are all effective treatment options. One key thing you can do is offer believable reassurance. Once you are sure your family member is not having a physical medical emergency, respond with a calm, steady voice and reassure him that he is not having a medical crisis.

Many people with anxiety find it helpful to do the deep breathing and relaxation exercises described in chapter 6. These will often help him calm down and feel better. In addition, some of the new medications used to treat mood disorders can effectively treat anxiety.

CHAPTER 2

Signs of Depression to Look For

If you think your spouse, child, parent, or friend might have depression or bipolar depression, there are some things to look for that will help your efforts to assist her. Watch for physical changes in the person, listen to the way she says she feels, and observe the way she acts. Look for changes in

- general appearance
- habits vital to functioning, like sleep and appetite (called *vital senses*)
- feelings and attitudes about herself
- thoughts about suicide

Pay attention if you notice any of these changes in your friend or family member. Use these observations as you try to gently encourage her to seek professional help. If she's an adolescent or an elderly person under your care, it can be quite helpful to report these changes to her primary care doctor or mental health providers.

General Appearance

Try to think about how your family member appears today in general:

Is she neat, clean, and well-groomed; sloppy and disheveled; or somewhere in between?

Is she alert and bright or dark and moody?

Most important, is she her usual baseline self? Is she sad or irritable in mood, speech, or facial expression?

Does she cry frequently?

Does she appear disinterested in her surroundings and the activities she's always liked? For example, has she stopped participating in her weekly aerobics class or monthly book club?

Watch for your family member spending excess time alone in her room or lying on the couch watching television or staring straight ahead. One characteristic of depression is a loss of interest in life and the activities she used to enjoy. These new behaviors may indicate illness.

Ask yourself if she appears tired and fatigued or slumped over in posture or if her movements are sluggish. Note if her speech is clear or slow and muffled. Depression saps the energy out of a person, and fatigue for no other clinical reason is something significant.

Notice whether your family member is taking care of herself—attending to self-care, bathing, grooming, and wearing clean clothes. Any deviation from her typical daily habits may signal depression.

Vital Senses, the Habits Vital to Our Functioning

Ask yourself if there has been any change from her usual behavior in the habits vital to daily functioning, such as sleep and appetite:

Has she gone into a pattern of sleeping more or less than usual?

Has she mentioned difficulty falling asleep, staying asleep, or waking up earlier than necessary?

Have you seen a change in her appetite or food habits?

Has she lost her usual amount of energy for daily life?

Note whether she takes a nap in the afternoon or early evening. Depression is often accompanied by a disruption in sleep patterns. This change could be a significant sign.

Does she eat more or less than usual? Is it the same type of food, or has she started eating junk food or fast food? This may indicate illness as well. Has this shift in appetite or dietary habits caused a change in her body weight, such as gaining or losing five pounds or more within 2 weeks? In some people, depression can lead to an unintentional (meaning the person did not deliberately lose or gain weight) change in body weight over time.

Do you have difficulty getting her up to go to school or work? Does she still participate in her previous physical exercise activities, such as aerobics class, jogging, or basketball? Any variation in these activities, when not related to a physical problem, may be a sign of depression.

Attitude about Self

Note if her feelings and attitudes about herself and her life have changed from her usual:

> Have her thoughts about herself and her experiences become negative and distorted?

> Has she expressed thoughts of worthlessness or guilt?

> Does she have difficulty thinking, concentrating, reading, or following a conversation or television show?

> Has she mentioned death or suicide?

> Does she express inaccurate and negative thoughts about herself, such as "I'm a loser" or "Nobody ever likes me"?

Biased, automatically negative thinking can frequently occur in depression. An overview in table 4.1 describes the different types of thought distortions common to depression. The information there may help you recognize distortions in thinking.

Think about whether your family member has mentioned any loss of hope for her future, school, job, career, or social opportunities. Hopelessness is a key feature of this illness in many people. So is a feeling of worthlessness, in which she ignores her positive qualities. Feeling guilty for something she had little or no control over is also worth noting. Has she mentioned having difficulty with thinking, concentrating, reading, or following a conversation or a show on television? Trouble with concentration and focus is the top symptom of depression self-reported on the Web site Patients Like Me (www.patientslikeme.com). Has she had any thoughts of death or suicide or even vaguely mentioned not wanting to "be around"? You will want to take any slight comment like this very seriously. Suicidal thoughts indicate that she requires immediate professional help.

Warning Signs of Suicide and Risk Factors for Suicide

The most severe form of depression can lead someone to consider suicide. This may or may not apply to your family member or friend at some point. Suicide is one of the greatest tragedies known to us. It claims approximately 41,000 lives each year in the United States (National Institute of Mental Health [NIMH] 2015). It is the second leading cause of death in those aged 15 to 34 (Centers for Disease Control [CDC] 2015). Suicidal thoughts and behaviors of any kind are considered a psychiatric emergency. They require immediate response.

The Warning Signs of Suicide (American Foundation for Suicide Prevention [AFSP] 2015) are listed in table 2.1. Warning Signs of Suicide are distinct changes in the things your family member or friend says, does, or thinks that are noticed by others. They include talking about death or suicide, having a suicide plan, feeling severe hopelessness, experiencing a drastic change in behavior, withdrawing from her normal activities, losing interest in people or social activities, and more. For example, she might mutter, "I wish I hadn't been born," "I'd be better off dead," or "Everybody would be better off without me." She might start giving away her prized possessions, withdraw from friends and family, or start to use or increase her use of alcohol or street drugs. Pay close attention to these statements and actions; consider them an alert that she's serious about harming herself.

Table 2.1. Warning Signs of Suicide

In talking

    Talks about killing self or having a suicide plan

    Believes he or she has no reason to live

    Concerned about being a burden to others

    Has unbearable emotional pain

In behavior

    Increased use of alcohol or drugs

    Looks for a way to kill self

    Acts recklessly

    Withdraws from activities and life

    Isolates self from family and friends

    Sleeps too much or too little

    Says goodbye to others

    Gives away possessions

    Behaves aggressively

In mood

    Depression

    Loss of interest

    Anger, rage, irritability

    Humiliation

    Anxiety

Source: According to the American Foundation for Suicide Prevention (AFSP, www.afsp.org) www.afsp.org/preventing-suicide-warning-signs, accessed July 2015.

Your first response when your family member or friend mentions harming herself is to sit down with her and discuss her feelings and thoughts on death and suicide. It can be very scary to hear about suicide and to talk about it. If you are unable to have this conversation, call for professional help immediately. If you feel you can speak about it, take a deep breath and stay calm during this conversation. You can be most helpful if you talk to your family member or friend about her thoughts of self-harm and any suicidal thoughts or plans she may have.

You could start by saying, "I've been very concerned about you lately. Have you ever thought about harming yourself or wishing that you weren't here?" Let her know you care and that she's not alone. Do your best to listen. Try to use words that are supportive, not judgmental or dismissive. For example, if she mentions thoughts of suicide, it's not helpful to quickly respond with, "No, you don't! How could you possibly think that way?" Instead, ask her directly and gently about the specific details of any suicide plans she might be considering, such as, "Do you have a plan?" and "Do you have what you need to carry out your plan?" If your family member shows any indication of suicide intent or a plan, your first step is to call for professional help immediately by dialing 9-1-1 or her mental health provider. In the meantime, remove anything (pills, knives, firearms) she might use for this purpose from her environment. Do not leave her alone.

Some people fear that speaking of suicide with someone who has depression may make the situation worse. But having this conversation will *not* encourage her to take action. Asking about suicide and encouraging your family member or friend to get help do not increase the risk of suicide (CDC 1992). Suicide is usually considered an impulsive action in a troubled person who sees no way to change her painful circumstances. She sees no way out. A suicidal act often surprises family members and close friends because the person is not perceived as impulsive and hides the emotional pain deep inside.

Some age groups may be more vulnerable to contemplating self-harm or suicide. Many teenagers have a difficult time during this phase of their lives. They feel pressure to succeed and fit in with their peers. Some struggle with self-esteem and self-doubt. This age group also exhibits a fair amount of impulsive behavior. Older adults may face loneliness, loss of friends and family, physical impairments that limit their lifestyle, medical problems and chronic pain, retirement, or loss of independence and purpose (Alpass et al. 2003). If your family member shows any signs of suicide intent, consider it an emergency and follow the steps outlined above.

There are some Risk Factors for Suicide that you should be aware of (CDC, National Suicide Prevention Lifeline). They could increase the chance that your loved one might consider or attempt suicide. The Risk Factors for Suicide only point out that a person has a higher likelihood for suicide based on her life history. They are not the same as the Warning Signs of Suicide, which are distinct changes in a person's behavior or speech. The Risk Factors for Suicide are listed in table 2.2. These include a previous suicide attempt, a family history of suicide, a history of trauma or abuse, a history of alcohol and substance abuse, hopelessness, male gender, living alone or in social isolation, and many others. They may or may not apply to your family member or friend.

Once you know the factors that put your family member or friend at risk, you can take the following steps to prevent suicide. First, ensure she receives effective medical care for her mental, physical, or substance use disorders with a combination of medical and mental health treatments. You may want to help her arrange these treatments since the telephone calls and paperwork to schedule appointments can be an effort. She may also need a referral for these treatments from her primary care physician, depending on her type of health insurance plan.

Second, make sure she has no access to lethal means of suicide: pills, firearms, knives, other weapons, etc. This means going

Table 2.2. Risk Factors for Suicide

The Risk Factors for Suicide are those parts of a person's history that may make the person more likely to harm himself or herself. These include:

» Mental disorders such as depression, bipolar disorder, anxiety, personality disorders, or schizophrenia
» Family history of suicide
» Previous suicide attempt
» Alcohol or substance abuse
» Male
» Single, divorced, widowed, or separated
» Teenage or elderly
» Living alone or socially isolated
» Unemployed
» Feelings of hopelessness
» Impulsive and aggressive tendencies
» History of trauma or abuse
» Chronic physical illness or chronic pain
» Major loss—job, financial, or relationship
» Easy access to lethal means (guns, weapons, pills, etc.)
» Lack of social support and social isolation
» Lack of health care
» Cultural and religious beliefs
» Local epidemics of suicides
» Stigma associated with seeking help

Additional References: National Alliance on Mental Illness (NAMI), www.nami.org; Centers for Disease Control and Prevention (CDC), www.cdc.gov/violenceprevention/suicide; National Suicide Prevention Lifeline, www.suicidepreventionlifeline.org/learn/riskfactors.

through the house from top to bottom and removing anything she might be able to use or that might tempt her or put her at risk.

Third, and most important, provide her with support and a strong connection to you, her friends and family, and her community. This includes support through her ongoing medical and mental health providers. Last, encourage her to learn and use skills in problem solving, resolving conflicts, and handling her problems in a nonviolent way. For many people, spiritual and religious beliefs that validate the need for self-preservation and discourage self-harm have been very useful.

CHAPTER 3

Support and Communication Strategies

In this book I walk you through some helpful things that you as a family member, significant other, or close friend can do for someone who is depressed. You will see that often, it's a matter of knowing just what to say or do in the moment. This can be easier said than done. So how do you know the most useful actions to take or words to say? The first thing to remember is that you—the family members and close friends—are the ones who provide daily support and encouragement, a very important element. You might then wonder what that support really involves. On an emotional level, "Support . . . involves time spent listening, hearing and acknowledging the emotions that the patient is experiencing, and also advocating on the patient's behalf" (Buckman 1992).

Providing Support

Providing support is a very good place for you to start. Although you may not realize it, giving support to someone who is ill is usually considered a huge job. It's an effort that can continue 24 hours a day. It may at times be difficult and result in your own burnout. It is important to take good care of yourself during this time so you remain better energized to care for your family member or friend. Chapter 8 of this book can help you with this.

The overall goal in providing emotional support is for your family member or friend to know that you are listening and interested in what he thinks. This is a very important message to get across to him. How do you best do this? Others in your situation find the following approach helpful. Focus your efforts on

- listening without judging
- hearing what he says
- responding with empathy to his words

An *empathic response* means that you try to identify with and understand your friend or family member's feelings or problems. One of the most common challenges you may find is a breakdown in listening (table 3.1 lists the causes of this). The rest of this chapter will offer effective listening and communication strategies.

You can provide other types of support as well, such as financial, physical, or household support. Everyone with depression has different needs, and caregivers have different abilities to assist in these areas. Each type of support you offer may be appropriate at the time depending on your family member or friend's age, personal circumstances, and extent of illness. For example, you may offer to accompany your elderly parent to a doctor's appointment, help a friend with grocery shopping, or take your cousin's dog to the vet. Your goal is to help without making your family member or friend feel entirely dependent. It's important that you

- be clear and consistent in what you can and cannot offer in support
- set clear limits and expectations for both you and your family member or friend
- try not to promise anything you cannot deliver

Communication Strategies

Your family member or friend may feel helped now if he knows you are consistently there for him. This means you try to regularly set aside a time and place for private conversation to check in on how he is doing. Do you feel awkward doing this? That's not uncommon—many people in your position do. But most people with depression actually find it helps to talk about it. Talking about it does not make the depression worse; your family member may be relieved to know that his depression symptoms make sense, have a name, and that his condition is common and legitimate. Try to show respect, dignity, and regard for his privacy in your words and actions. Make your best effort to accept what he says. Don't repeat anything he tells you in confidence unless it is a threat to his life and safety or that of others.

Here's a suggestion for what you can do now: sit down with your family member or friend and encourage him to speak openly, in his own words. Let him express his feelings and emotions without interruption. This will show him that his feelings and experiences are important. However, try to understand that someone who has depression is not always able or willing to talk about his feelings or what he privately discussed in therapy. You might feel shut out, but it's usually not intended personally.

In this conversation, show that you have *heard* what he said. The following steps may help guide you (Buckman 1992):

Prepare. Use open body language, which means making your best effort to do as many of the following as you can: sit down; remain calm; relax your posture without folding your arms, pointing your finger, or fidgeting; turn your body toward your family member or friend; give him your full attention and shut off your cell phone; make eye contact; and use a clear, calm voice.

Use active listening. This way of communicating tells him you are fully present and paying attention to what he is saying. It's not easy to do, especially if your mind tends to wander. If that happens, try to bring it right back to the topic. It gets easier to do with practice. Active listening is important to try because it often helps you to build rapport, understanding, and trust. It can help you avoid misunderstandings and frequently enables your family member or friend to open up. To actively listen, try the following:

- Focus on his words without allowing your mind to stray.
- Use open body language to show you are listening and interested.

- Make eye contact.
- Let him speak without interruption.
- Encourage him to talk by nodding your head and saying, "Tell me more" or "Um-hmm."
- Respond periodically by restating, reflecting, or summarizing (see below) his words.
- Ask open questions to draw him out, such as, "How did that make you feel?" or "What do you think would happen if . . ."
- Tolerate short periods of silence. This can be difficult. He may be silent if his feelings are very intense or if he's deep in thought. Accept that for the moment. A short period of silence often gives him permission to feel or express his emotions. Occasionally, break the silence by asking, "What were you thinking of just now?"

Show that you have *heard* him: this indicates that you understand what he has said and that his words have meaning. In this way you may be able to validate his feelings. You don't have to agree with him. Try to respond to him in one of the following ways:

- Repeat his exact words (repetition).
- Repeat what he says in your own words (paraphrase).
- Identify and state the emotion his words suggest (reflection). Reflection effectively shows you have both heard and interpreted what he said. For example, if he says, "Life is no good. It's never going to change for me," you might respond with, "I hear that life feels no good to you right now and seems hopeless." This acknowledges his feelings and sense of hopelessness. It is important to interpret his words as accurately as possible. Otherwise, you might lose the trust you've just worked to build. If you are unsure about the emotion he is feeling, avoid using the reflection response.

You can also show that you have heard your family member or friend by periodically summarizing what he says. This allows you to clarify what was said and lets him expand further on his thoughts. For example, you might say:

It appears that _____.
It sounds like _____.
What you seem to be saying is _____.
Is that the case? Do I understand correctly?

Ask questions. Questions are a great way to show interest and clarify facts so that you understand the point your family member or friend is trying to make. You can ask different types of questions in conversation; each may have a different impact on someone in distress. Some examples include:

- Closed question. A *closed question* is designed to obtain a specific answer. It allows only a few potential responses such as yes or no. It doesn't give your family member or friend a chance to express his feelings and emotions or describe a stressful situation. An example of a closed question is, "Did your doctor renew your prescription today?" (yes or no). Try to use this type of question sparingly.
- Open question. An *open question* allows your family member or friend to respond in any way he chooses. It gives him permission to talk openly about his feelings or experiences. An example of an open question would be, "How did that make you feel?," or "What did you make of that?" Try to use open questions often to learn more about what your family member may be feeling and why.

Respond. You may find several good ways of responding to your family member or friend in the course of a conversation. You can make a nonjudgmental statement (repeat, paraphrase, or reflect), use body language such as a head nod, ask an open question, or be silent for a short period. Of these, the most effective response is often an empathic response, a type of reflection.

How do you provide an empathic response? To begin, try to

identify the emotion your family member or friend may be feeling, such as sadness, anxiety, or fear. Then think about where that emotion came from, such as from a previous experience. Next, do your best to put them both together and respond in a way that shows you understand the connection between the two. For example, if he is upset about not being able to participate on the track team because of his illness, you might say, "You sound really sad about missing the track season this year and not being able to compete with your team because of your depression." This shows him that you both hear and understand his distress. In this way you have identified his emotion (sad) and where it came from (missing the track season as a result of his depression).

Or, in another example, if he is distraught and says that nobody likes him, your most effective response could be to say something like, "It must be really awful to feel unlovable when your friends don't call." You have identified his emotion (awful and unlovable) and its source (because his friends don't call). One word of caution. Use this technique only if you really think you know what he's feeling—don't guess, as that attempt often backfires.

Listening is considered an art. As you practice, you generally improve at it. This is true for most people. Be aware of the ways we all can unconsciously block effective listening, and make your best effort to avoid them. Blocks to effective listening include making assumptions without knowing the facts, mindreading what the other person is thinking, making judgments, filtering out pieces of information (avoiding hearing some of the details), or daydreaming. Blocks to effective listening are described in table 3.1.

If your friend or family member appears angry or hostile during your conversation, it is generally not helpful to respond in a similar manner. That can often escalate the situation. It may also add to your own personal stress. Instead, try to stay calm, step back, and show that you recognize the source of his anger and emotions. Again, do this only if you think you understand the source of his anger—don't guess here. Making incorrect assumptions about his thoughts or feelings may only fuel his anger. If you think you know, you might say something like, "It must make you feel angry to lose a position on your team this year." This identifies his emotion, lets him know you understand his loss, and allows him the opportunity to respond.

Many things can cause your family member or friend to feel angry when he is ill with any prolonged medical problem, including an episode of depression (Buckman 1992). He could be angry with his personal situation and having his life turned upside down by depression. He might be trying to cope with changes in his daily routine away from work, school, friends, or colleagues; a change in his financial status; or a change in his recreational opportunities. He could be upset at having to deal with a mental illness or

Table 3.1. Blocks to Effective Listening

> » Making assumptions (without the facts)
> » Mind reading (when you conclude you know what someone is thinking without the facts)
> » Filtering out what he's saying (for example, when you avoid hearing some of the details)
> » Judging what someone is saying
> » Changing the subject to yourself or another topic
> » Comparing his experience to someone else's
> » Identifying (when you refer back to your own similar experience)
> » Rehearsing (when you focus on what you're going to say next)
> » Daydreaming or not paying attention
> » Giving advice
> » Sparring, put-downs, sarcasm, or debating a point
> » Needing to be right at any cost
> » Placating the person

Table 3.2. Anger in Your Family Member or Friend

Your family member or friend may feel angry with himself, you, others, or outside forces. He may believe any or all have negatively influenced him or his illness. The source may be inappropriate, and he may have no basis for such hostility. It may not seem rational to you as an observer. It is important, however, to understand what is behind his fury. Here is a list of potential targets for his anger:

Anger against the illness

He may feel anger at his symptoms, being disabled by the illness, the loss of freedom to do as he pleases, or the unfairness of it all (why me?).

Anger against his loss of control and lack of power

He may be angry because of his inability to control his life. He may feel overly dependent on friends, family, and his medical team.

Anger against his perceived loss of potential

He may feel anger because he believes his future hopes and dreams are lost.

Anger against himself

He may be angry with himself if he believes he caused his own illness. He may feel betrayed by his body and angry at his own negative attitude.

Anger against friends and family

He may resent the fact that friends and family enjoy good health. He may still be angry as a result of old family arguments. He may hate receiving advice, charity, and sympathy from others. He may believe that friends or family contributed to his illness, whether appropriate or inappropriate. He may feel angry and abandoned when he feels others are withdrawing from him.

Anger against medical and other health professional teams

He may blame his health care team for any news regarding his diagnosis, treatment, and outcome. He may feel he's given up control to his doctors or resent the perceived good health of his medical team. He may feel angry if he believes his mental health providers are cold, insensitive, or do not listen. He may be angry if there are communication gaps or he is not part of the decision making process, or does not agree with their decisions.

Anger against "outside forces"

He may be angry with his workplace situation (whether appropriately or inappropriately) or angry with his daily environment at home.

Anger against God

He may feel anger if he thinks that God or the divine has abandoned him. He may believe that God is unjustly punishing him. He may think that after all his years of keeping faith and religious observances, he is seeing a poor return on his efforts.

Source: Adapted from Robert Buckman, *How to Break Bad News: A Guide for Health Care Professionals* (Johns Hopkins University Press, 1992), 138–39.

angry with himself, his health care providers, you because you are there, a family member who doesn't understand his struggles, or an employer for letting him go. Table 3.2 provides examples of what could cause his anger response. Also, realize that during depression episodes some people, such as adult men or adolescents, may react more readily with irritability and anger instead of a low mood.

And keep in mind the following important point: wait until your family member's concerns have been stated and heard before you offer any reassuring words (such as "Everything will be okay"). If you do so too early, he might perceive it as a brush-off and may feel that his concerns are not valid.

CHAPTER 4

Helpful Approaches

As you approach your family member or friend who has depression, try to follow the suggestions in this chapter. They have helped many people just like you and her. They are offered in addition to the communication and support strategies that were described in chapter 3. Because following these suggestions may involve changing how you interact with someone, you might consider trying these approaches one at a time before adding a second and then a third. You will see they often make a difference.

To begin, do your best to treat your family member normally, which means making an effort to include her in your usual everyday activities and family and social plans. Make it clear that you expect her to participate in pleasurable activities as well as share in the daily chores around the house and keep up with responsibilities at school or work. She does not want to feel left out or different because of her illness. Let her be the one to determine if it's too much to handle. Help her modify her activities as needed, but try not to give her an easy out.

If she needs to take a leave of absence from work or school, do your best to treat it as a temporary setback, not a failure. You can expect her to slowly get back on track as her depression lifts. Many people with depression find their moods slowly lift as they make contact with others. This isn't always the case, however. Some people end up feeling worse after they see friends or family doing well and enjoying their lives.

In some cases you may need to set limits on your family member or friend's daily behavior. This may be difficult for both of you. Try to see that she understands you expect her to abide by the rules of the household or social group. You might even have to encourage her to bathe, style her hair, and wear clean clothes. Since it's important that a person who has depression not isolate herself from others, try to get her to share dinner each night with the family or social group.

In some cases you may also need to set expectations on how she relates with other family members or friends. Depression or bipolar disorder does not give anyone the right to be overly argumentative or demanding of others' time and patience. Try to let her know you expect her to act calmly, with courtesy and good manners toward other family members and friends, no matter how down, irritable, or bad she feels. You may need to specify boundaries on specific behaviors, curfews, and the use of alcohol and street drugs. For example, if your family member begins to indulge in late-night drinking binges, you will want to let her know that this is not healthy or acceptable. You may need to both clearly agree on what time she is expected home every evening and how she spends her free time. This is particularly important for young adults and adolescents. Try to make your expectations clear and stick to them. This can be a source of conflict in some families. If she resists or rebels, your best strategy may be to remain firm. Try to avoid giving in just because of her illness.

Try to Provide Hope

There is no medicine like hope, no incentive so great and no tonic so powerful as the expectation of something better tomorrow.
—Orison Swett Marden, founder, *Success* magazine

Often in depression, a person loses hope for herself, her future, and her world. It can be incapacitating. Your words and example can indicate that you have not lost hope for her—that you have expectations for her future and believe things will improve. This can be a powerful message. How do you convey it?

One way is to try to keep her plans for the future alive in conversation, even if those plans have to be modified for now. For example, if she has to take a leave of absence from work or school, you could say, "I expect that next fall when you get back to work [school, team, or committee] you'll be able to _____." She may feel encouraged on hearing that you expect she will successfully return to her usual activities. Your goal is to treat displaced plans as temporary setbacks, not failures.

If she lacks hope or optimism, try to suggest she "borrow" hope from someone who cares for her and believes she has potential. That person could be you. You might say, "I sense that you don't feel hopeful about _____ right now, but I do. Why don't you let me keep hope alive for you?" Through your eyes she may begin to see the possibilities in her life return. It may be difficult for you to maintain a positive, upbeat attitude when you too are struggling and all else seems grim. Try to focus on the fact that this is a treatable biological illness with ups and downs.

Next, do your best to set realistic expectations for your family member or friend. Convey to her that *right now* she may not be able to do everything she used to do—and that's okay. Right now she may have to modify her plans and responsibilities. This is often related to the depression and improves for most people. Your family member may feel validated knowing you don't believe she's weak or a failure or that she's lazy or "faking it." Try to accept what she can do now and encourage her to stretch her wings as she is able. For example, you might gently suggest she get involved in a hobby or activity she once enjoyed or return to work or school part-time, at a pace she can handle now.

It can be particularly helpful to show realistic optimism (Reivich and Shatte 2002; Southwick and Charney 2012). *Realistic optimism* is a reasonable view of the future that involves hope and the confidence that things will turn out well, with enough hard work and determination. It means discussing her realistic plans for the future and supporting her efforts to get there.

If your family member or friend has had more than one episode of depression in her life, try not to assume she will automatically know how to handle the next one. This isn't realistic. It often takes a lot of time, effort, and skill working with a mental health professional for someone who has depression to successfully manage her illness. For example, it may require a great deal of insight and practice on her part to anticipate the triggers; handle the difficult times of life, such as dreaded holidays or certain relationships; and take the steps to minimize their effects. This can be frustrating to you as an observer. Patience and understanding are essential.

The next approach is to try to help her confront negative thoughts. It is very common for those who have depression to see themselves and the world through a negative lens they strongly believe is accurate. This means that everything she sees, thinks, and believes automatically has a negative twist or bias to it. These *automatic negative thoughts* are extreme distortions in thinking and overwhelm a person's reasoning (Beck et al. 1979).

Common negative thoughts include, "I'm a loser," "I can't do anything right," "Nobody likes me," "Everybody hates me," or "I always drop the ball." The different types of automatic negative thoughts are listed in table 4.1. They are usually repetitive, not necessarily logical or based on fact, and can seem frustrating from your point of view. Examples include black-and-white or all-or-nothing thinking, filtering (filtering out the positive and focusing only on the negative), jumping to conclusions, or catastrophizing (Burns 2009). You don't have to fully understand the different types of thought distortions in this list. Just know that they are possibilities and that someone with depression may unintentionally think this way.

You may help your family member or friend greatly by gently encouraging her to challenge those negative thought distortions. Although some family members fear that talking about it may make things worse, that's not usually the case. You can try this now using one or more of the following suggestions. They are not meant for you to act as her therapist. She may or may not be willing or able to discuss these issues with you on any given day.

Table 4.1. Types of Distorted Thinking

Distortions in thinking, called cognitive distortions, are common in depression. Your family member or friend's perception of an event can be twisted or inaccurate in some of the following ways:

Filtering: focusing on and magnifying the negative details while ignoring (filtering out) the positive in a situation. A person will reject or minimize good experiences and insist they "don't count."

Polarized or all-or-nothing thinking: thinking at one extreme or the other, in black or white, good or bad categories. For example, if someone cooks a meal that isn't perfect, she sees herself as a total failure, the worst extreme.

Overgeneralizing: making a general conclusion based on a single event or piece of evidence. If something bad happens, a person expects it to occur over and over again. She sees a single negative event as permanent and often uses the words "always" and "never."

Global labeling: generalizing one or two qualities into an overall negative judgment and applying a label. It's an extreme form of overgeneralization. For example, someone might label herself a "loser" based on one less-than-perfect behavior.

Jumping to conclusions: immediately interpreting something in a negative way without having the facts.

Mind reading: concluding that she knows what others are feeling, why they act a certain way, or how they feel, without their saying so.

Fortune telling: believing she knows how future events will turn out without any supporting evidence.

Catastrophizing: expecting the worst, a disaster. This type of thinking often includes the "What ifs . . ."

Minimizing: discounting the positive aspects of herself or her actions and insisting they "don't count."

Personalizing: thinking that everything people say or do is a reaction to her personally. Or, she assumes total responsibility and blames herself for an event out of her control.

Blaming: holding others responsible for her pain or alternatively, blaming herself for every problem.

Emotional reasoning: believing that what she feels must automatically be true. For example, if she "feels" stupid then she must be stupid.

Being right: being continually defensive and having to prove that her feelings, opinions, and actions are right. Being wrong is unthinkable.

Reward fallacy: expecting that all of her sacrifice and self-denial will pay off. And feeling bitter and resentful when it doesn't happen.

Source: Adapted in part from David Burns, *Feeling Good: The New Mood Therapy* (HarperCollins, 2009), table 3.1, 42–43.

- Help her replace automatic negative thoughts with alternative, more realistic thoughts. If she says, "Nobody likes me. I have no friends," you might gently ask her to really think about where that thought comes from. Suggest she replace it with something accurately reflecting her life today. You might say, "I hear you feel like you are unlovable and have no friends. That must feel awful. Where do you think that comes from? What about the people in your book club? Didn't you tell me some of them like you?" Let her be the one to come up with the alternative thought, such as, "Well, I do have a few friends in my book club." Then ask if she feels better after this exercise. Often, this is the case.

- When negative thoughts surface in your family member or friend who has depression, try this exercise: Start by having her focus on a particular negative thought. She will need a piece of paper with two columns, one titled "Evidence FOR" the thought and one titled "Evidence AGAINST" the thought. Have her consider the evidence in her life *against* the negative thought and the evidence *for* the negative thought and fill in the two columns. See the example in table 4.2. If she has trouble, she may need to ask friends or family for suggestions. Many people with depression find more evidence against the negative thought than for it. Seeing this, your family member or friend may realize the error of her thinking. This may help to lift her mood.

- Try to challenge negative thoughts by asking your family member or friend to remember her past successes. If she believes she's a failure, as many people with depression do, she will probably deny ever having any past successful outcomes. The negative thoughts in depression often cause a person to believe she has failed in life, is incompetent, or is a loser. Point out her achievements, whether in school, work, sports, or a hobby. For example, you might ask, "What about the time you were recognized at work for your big project?," or "Remember the time you won a blue ribbon in the 5K road race?" With real-life evidence before her, denial becomes more difficult. She may push aside those negative beliefs and accept some degree of competence in herself.

- Ask your family member or friend how she successfully dealt with a tough situation in the past. She may initially deny ever having overcome adversity. Try to use gentle persuasion to remind her of those events. You could say, "I remember the time you had a difficult project to do and you _____ ," or "What about the time when _____ happened and you were able to _____?" Recognizing these successes may boost her self-confidence and eventually her mood.

- Try to get your family member or friend to explore what's behind her negative thoughts. Where and when did they start? Ask her whether the issues underlying these thoughts are current and bother her now or if they are from years past. For example, you might ask, "Are you just now thinking about _____ [negative thought]? Did this come up recently, or have you been thinking about it for a while? How does it affect you now?" Past experiences can often haunt someone who has depression. Thinking about them constantly, called *rumination*, is both common and unhelpful. Ask her what's in her power to try to change now. Encourage her to put aside negative thoughts stemming from the past. This could bring her a great deal of relief.

Watch for Warning Signs of Depression

A number of people who experience depression or bipolar disorder exhibit warning signs that become obvious just before their depression or mania worsens. Warning signs are distinct changes from the person's usual thoughts, feelings, behaviors, actions, daily routines, or self-care habits. You may notice them right before a decline in mood. Warning signs can include:

Table 4.2. Evidence For and Against

When a thought, belief, or interpretation of an event causes you distress, it's helpful to examine the evidence for and against it. This will help you identify and change thoughts based on inaccurate assumptions.

Step 1. Identify a negative or distressing thought.

Step 2. Gather evidence for and against that thought.

» Collect specific evidence about the thought to check its accuracy.

» Ask others who know you well for their realistic, honest feedback about the thought.

» Seek out experiences that counteract your negative beliefs. For example, go out and do some activity and observe what really happens. You will see first-hand the evidence against them.

Step 3. Look at your list realistically and see where the evidence lies.

Ask yourself: Is your belief inherently true, or is it an internalized message from your environment? If you find it is true, think about what is in your power to change.

Belief or thought	Evidence for ...	Evidence against ...

Source: Susan J. Noonan, *Managing Your Depression: What You Can Do to Feel Better* (Johns Hopkins University Press, 2013), 99–100.

- More negative thoughts
- More feelings of hopelessness, sadness, irritability, anxiety, or fatigue
- Appetite loss
- Sleep disruption
- Changes in personal hygiene, such as failure to bathe
- Difficulty with daily routines
- Loss of interest in previously enjoyed activities
- Excessive alcohol use
- Slipping grades in school

Each person has a characteristic, unique pattern of warning signs. Sometimes, these are subtle. Try to learn about and look for your family member or friend's particular type and pattern of warning signs. If you notice anything, that is the time to encourage the call for professional help and follow the Basics of Mental Health outlined later in this chapter. Recognizing her warning signs early may give you the chance to step in and try to change the course of her depression or bipolar episode. The following story of Jan and David shows the subtle warning signs of depression that you need to pay attention to.

Jan is just beside herself. She's been married to David for 15 years. Together, they have two children, ages 9 and 11. Jan works outside the home half-time, and David works full time as a computer programmer, a job he enjoyed until the past few months. Since then he's been coming home from work irritable and solemn, reluctant to speak to Jan about any issues going on at work. This is unlike him. She doesn't know if anything happened, but she guesses David is upset about work-related budget constraints, tight deadlines, and a boss who's been particularly critical lately. But she's not sure because David clams up and won't talk to her.

Instead, he takes it out on her and the kids, finding fault with the way she cooks, the kids' behavior, the house—just about anything. He has stopped jogging and working out, activities he always enjoyed, and refuses to take the children to their soccer games and birthday parties. His best friend and brother have called to speak with him a few times and he won't take their calls. He says he's "too tired."

Several times, Jan has found David up in the middle of the night, unable to sleep, drinking a few beers (he says beer isn't *really* alcohol) or scotch. Lately, he's taken to having a scotch or two right when he gets home at night. One day Jan found a bottle of half-opened vodka hidden in his workroom. When she expressed her concern and suggested he visit their family doctor, David snapped at her and told her to leave him alone.

Jan is concerned for their children and doesn't want them to see David's behavior or ride in the car with him. She is planning to remove all alcohol from the house. Jan is persistent and plans to get his brother and best friend to sit down with him. She hopes they can get him to open up and agree to see his doctor.

As you can see, David is showing the warning signs of being more withdrawn and less communicative than usual and is isolating himself from his brother and friends. He is irritable and has trouble sleeping. He has stopped exercising and taking his children to their activities, things he previously enjoyed. Last, he has started drinking alcohol, privately and in front of his family. In response, Jan is considering removing all alcohol from the house. She also plans to have his friends talk to him and try to convince him to seek professional help.

The Basics of Mental Health

Just like the rest of our body, the brain needs continued care to function well. The most effective way to do this is by trying to follow a set of daily self-help steps called the Basics of Mental Health (Noonan 2013). These are the essentials we are all advised to do to maintain emotional health and stability. They include maintaining a regular pattern of sleep, diet, exercise, medications, routine and structure, and contact with friends.

Your family member or friend may find them challenging to do while dealing with the symptoms of a mood disorder. The symptoms of depression or bipolar disorder often interfere with one's ability to follow the Basics. However, these steps do help to improve the symptoms of depression. Sound scientific information supports this (Bodnar and Wisner 2005; Dunn et al. 2005; Frank 2007; Jacka et al. 2010; Mead et al. 2009; Rethorst and Trivedi 2013; Trivedi et al. 2006; Tsuno, Besset, and Ritchie 2005; Yeung, Feldman, and Fava 2010). They take hard work and perseverance to follow when depressed, but the results are worth it.

You can take on the role of coach and gently encourage her to stick to these Basics. You may choose to adopt a few of these healthy guidelines for yourself. In so doing you become an example of a healthy lifestyle for your family member or friend. Doing the Basics together with you may make it easier for her to follow them. This means that you try to keep regular sleep hours yourself, prepare nutritious meals for the family, and don't stock junk foods in the kitchen. You might offer to join your family member or friend for a walk or bike ride outdoors, encourage her to connect with other friends and family, and help her keep to a routine and daily structure by getting her an agenda book to plan daily activities.

The Basics of Mental Health

- Treat any physical illness.
- Sleep
  - Aim for 7 to 8 hours of sleep each night.

- Go to bed and wake up at the same time every day of the week, including non-work and non-school days.
- Keep your sleep environment quiet and relaxing.
- Reserve the bed for sleep only and no other activities such as eating, working, reading, watching television, etc.
- Track your sleep routine with a Sleep Diary and share it with your doctor.
- Follow the Sleep Hygiene guidelines to promote restful sleep, as outlined in table 6.3.
- Diet and nutrition
  - Eat three healthy, balanced meals each day.
  - Avoid street drugs and alcohol.
  - Limit caffeine intake.
  - For basic nutritional guidelines see www.choosemyplate.gov and Dietary Guidelines for Americans in table 6.2.
- Medications
  - Take all medications as prescribed.
  - Talk to your doctor about using vitamins and herbal supplements.
- Exercise regularly
  - Seek a balance of cardiovascular, strength training, and stretch/relaxation activities 3 to 5 days per week.
  - Strive for 150 minutes of moderate exercise per week or 75 minutes of vigorous exercise per week (U.S. Department of Health and Human Services [HHS] Physical Activity Guidelines for Americans 2008).
- Maintain positive social contact with your friends and family on a regular basis. Try to avoid isolation.
- Have a routine and structure to each day
  - Structure your time each day.
  - Write your daily tasks and appointments in an agenda book.
  - Break large tasks into small steps.
  - Include positive, pleasurable experiences in your day as well as home, family, and work responsibilities.

You might wonder how and why these Basics have an impact on your family member or friend's mood and depression symptoms. That's a very good question. Sleep is essential for all of us to function well. We all need sleep to restore and repair the effects of the day. Sleep problems often occur during an episode of depression or bipolar disorder. Your family member or friend may sleep too much, too little, or in fragmented bursts. If manic, she may be energized and require little sleep. Normally, adults require, on average, 7 to 8 hours per night of uninterrupted sleep.

Without enough sleep, your family member may become irritable, fatigued, or have trouble with concentration. Sound sleep optimizes brain function and is thought to have a positive effect on mood, so it follows that a change in sleep can affect depression. *Sleep Hygiene* refers to the personal habits and environmental conditions (what it's like in your bedroom) that affect your sleep. It's important for everyone, but especially those who have mood disorders, to keep good sleep habits and a consistent sleeping pattern in a bedroom that favors sound sleep.

Food is the fuel that keeps our brains and bodies operating properly. If a person skips meals or relies on unhealthy choices, junk food, or illegal drugs, the brain does not function well, leading to physical and mental fatigue and irritability. A poor or irregular diet may make your family member or friend vulnerable to depression. A Mediterranean diet high in fruits, vegetables, grains, beans, fish, poultry, and olive oil is often recommended (Jacka et al. 2010; Mayo Clinic 2015; Sanchez-Villegas et al. 2009). It is associated with a lower rate of depression.

For help with healthy meal preparation, the United States Department of Agriculture (USDA) has an easy-to-follow interactive Web site at www.choosemyplate.gov with information about balanced meals and healthy portion sizes. In addition, the HHS and the USDA jointly publish dietary guidelines for healthy eating (www.dietaryguidelines.gov). These are included in table 6.2.

The *Dietary Guidelines 2010* now display healthy food as portions divided on a dinner plate with fruits, vegetables, grains, lean protein, and a small amount of dairy. The guidelines recommend that half your plate be fruits and vegetables or that you eat five half-cup servings of colorful fruits and vegetables each day. For adults, the protein portion should be five to six ounces of lean meat, poultry, fish, or eggs daily. Grains should be three ounces per serving. Dairy should be low fat and used in moderation. The USDA also has an online tool to plan, analyze, and track your diet and physical activity, called the SuperTracker (www.supertracker.usda.gov). It can help your family member or friend with goal setting, virtual coaching, and journaling.

Regular physical exercise is equally important to the brain's function. It may counteract the sense of fatigue that comes along with depression. Exercise releases certain chemicals in the brain in addition to the "feel-good" *endorphins*. These chemicals, called *brain derived neurotrophic factor* (BDNF), act like fertilizer for the brain and promote the growth of new brain cells. Exercise improves mood and is considered helpful in depression and bipolar disorder. Your family member or friend can be helped by doing a combination of aerobic activities that increase her heart rate and breathing; strength training that builds and maintains bones and muscle; and balance and stretching activities such as yoga, tai chi, or stretching.

Those who have depression tend to isolate themselves, withdrawing from their usual activities and their friends and family. Your family member or friend may prefer to stay at home, stop answering the phone, and stay in her pajamas all day. It's a huge effort to get out and interact with people. Social isolation can have a big impact on mood, however, driving it down. Try to push her a little and encourage her to get out and see people and do the things she used to enjoy. Keeping up with social contacts may help maintain emotional well-being and protect against depression.

Empty hours of unscheduled or alone time frequently worsen the symptoms of depression. Having routine and structure to one's day can counteract the overwhelming impact of some symptoms like lethargy, fatigue, and loss of interest in activities. It's important that your family member or friend try to have a routine and schedule her day, without being rigid. She may find it easy to use a paper or electronic agenda that she can carry around and refer to frequently. She could include in it her work and home responsibilities, daily self-care, physical exercise schedule, social contacts, and positive experiences. It is most useful if she keeps it prioritized, with a timeframe and specific items that are attainable and realistic. Doing this may provide a sense of accomplishment and of being in control of her life.

Set Boundaries

You may find that a person who has depression or bipolar disorder can occasionally be difficult to live with. Her behavior may distress you and others in your family or social group. She may be upset, irritable, or very sad. She may not think clearly and take her feelings out on you and others.

As this book makes clear, it is important to understand what depression is. It's also important, however, to "use your understanding of the illness to cope, not to excuse" unacceptable behavior (Sheffield 1998). Family life will be easier and of higher quality if you set boundaries when needed. *Boundaries* are rules or limits on behavior that are agreed upon by you and the person who has depression. They provide a feeling of safety for your family member when things feel out of control. Work with her to set these boundaries in a firm but compassionate way.

Here's how you might go about doing it: Together, you both agree beforehand about what will be considered problematic or socially unacceptable behavior. This is generally not an easy conversation. Your family member may give you a hard time and be unwilling to go along. Your best approach is to be firm and consistent. You might begin by defining what behavior you will or will not tolerate. For example, you might specify limits on late-night activities, alcohol or illegal substance use, or a lack of self-care such as failing to bathe. Try to be very clear about what the consequences for misbehavior will be; follow through with them consistently if there is a breach. Here are some examples of boundaries you may want to include in your agreement (Sheffield 1998):

1. *Compliance with treatment and medication.* For any number of reasons, your family member may stop taking her psychiatric medications. These drugs can make her groggy or nauseated or have other side effects. She may worry that her friends or employer will judge her harshly if they know she takes medication.

People who have depression or bipolar disorder may get fed up with all of the talk therapy (*psychotherapy*) sessions they are required to attend. Talking about life events and intimate feelings can be hard. It brings up strong emotions. Traveling to sessions, keeping track of schedules, filling out insurance paperwork, paying medical bills—all can lead someone to drop a session or two or decide to quit therapy entirely.

Stopping medications and talk therapy can interfere with recovery and well-being. A team approach is often most effective to help convince someone to continue treatment. It is most effective if you, other family members, and her health care provider work together to encourage her cooperation with her treatment plan. Try to find out what caused her to stop the medications and see if you can help her solve that issue. Remind her that consistency with medications and treatment may often help her achieve the goals she so strongly desires. Use whatever means available to get her to agree to the overall treatment plan.

2. *Tough love.* Your family member's behavior may be so trying that you need to apply a tough love approach. Perhaps she is extremely argumentative, angry, abusive, or hurting herself or friends or other family members. Use the tough love tactic to stay firm while loving.

Tough love is a method in which your troubled child or teen sees your love for her while you apply a firm and consistent approach in discipline, expectations, boundaries, and limits and follow through on the consequences of misbehavior as appropriate. In this model your teen or young adult is responsible for her behavior, makes choices, and is held accountable for her (bad) choices.

For example, you might communicate that you will stop helping her until she clearly indicates she is willing to help herself. Or you might take privileges away from your rebellious teenager until she can show you she is able to comply with treatment and care for herself safely.

3. *Verbal abuse.* A person with depression or bipolar disorder may become so irritable and agitated that she feels and appears out of control. You may have to establish boundaries or rules against verbal outbursts of anger, insults, and verbal abuse toward you and other family members. Send her a clear message that you will not tolerate this kind of behavior. Setting boundaries may help her regain some control over her emotions. Deep down, she will thank you for it.

4. *Physical abuse.* Setting boundaries around physical abuse is a must. Never tolerate this type of behavior. Hitting, punching a wall, fist fighting, breaking objects, or other forms of violence may be your family member's way to express her frustration or anger. She does not know how else to express her emotions. That is not an excuse for bad behavior.

5. *Manipulation.* Some people with depression engage in subtle games of manipulation to get their own way. Your family member may attempt to look or sound helpless or incompetent so you or others will do things for her. Do not buy in to this. Despite her depression and bipolar disorder, she may still be capable of doing many things for herself. Try not to do for her what she is capable of doing for herself. Set expectations with her about what you will and will not do.

Zach's story below illustrates the difficulty of identifying the warning signs of depression in a teenager. You might not be sure if your family member is in a phase of adolescent behavior or if this is an indication of illness. This example shows that setting limits on daily behavior with a tough love approach can be a useful and responsible step for parents to take.

Jeff and Maria have a teenage son, Zach, age 17; an older daughter away at college; and a younger son in middle school. Zach is the middle child. Zach has always been an overachieving student and a skilled athlete, with a number of hobbies—until the past 4 months.

Maria noticed that his grades were slipping and that when asked he seemed not to care, which is highly unusual. One day Jeff received a phone call from Zach's basketball coach. Zach had missed too many practices and would be put on athletic probation. Jeff was shocked because Zach had led them to believe he was at practice. Now Jeff wondered what his son was doing with his time. So Jeff approached Zach, who told him to "bug off" and leave him alone. This kind of irritability is unusual for Zach. Maria and Jeff also noticed that Zach no longer hung out with his old crowd of friends from school. Kids would call the house and he wouldn't take their calls, or he'd respond to them with one-word answers.

He seemed to have a new group of friends, the "tough" kids that Maria was wary of. Rumor said they used alcohol and drugs. Was Zach into this too? They weren't sure. He came home drunk a few times. Was this normal teenage behavior or something else? He stayed out late, even on school nights, even though he had a 10:00 p.m. curfew during the week.

When home, Zach just moped around, avoiding family activities or conversation. He seemed sad. This was getting tough. Jeff and Maria tried to sit and talk to Zach on several occasions, but he was essentially mute. He refused to speak with anyone else, such as their family doctor or clergyman, whom he'd always admired. Jeff was worried about Zach and took the car keys away from him. This was out of concern for his safety and to prevent any reckless behavior. Jeff also hoped that this would motivate Zach to open up to them.

In this story Zach shows the warning signs of depression in a teenager: his school grades are slipping, he's irritable, he has a new group of friends, he's drinking alcohol, and he's staying out beyond his curfew, all of which his parents cannot control. In addition, he's been secretive about his whereabouts while failing to attend basketball practice. These behaviors are more than the usual teenage "acting out." Jeff and Maria attempted to speak with him, to no avail. They set boundaries with a curfew and adopted a tough love approach by taking his car keys away. This move was also for his personal safety, to keep him from drinking and driving.

Mental Health First Aid

An additional set of helpful tools is called First Aid for Depression, a movement for families and friends that began in Australia in 2001 (Langlands et al. 2008). It describes the Mental Health First Aid program as "the help provided to a person who has a mental health problem or is in a mental health crisis . . . given until appropriate professional treatment is received or the crisis resolves" (Kitchener and Jorm 2002; Langlands et al. 2008). The concept is to train family members, friends, and other responders to know what to look for and how to respond in an urgent mental health situation. It is similar in concept to CPR classes that train people to respond to someone in the midst of a medical emergency.

These intervention strategies are taught in training programs created by Mental Health First Aid Australia (MHFA), a national nonprofit charity focused on mental health training and research. The organization provides interesting and effective ways to respond to a person's depression. You can access their guidelines at www.mhfa.com.au. In the United States, a similar intervention project can be reviewed at www.mentalhealthfirstaid.org. Its goal is to provide free courses in prevention and early intervention. It is available to the general public. The course content teaches you the skills to

- assess the risk of suicide or harm
- listen nonjudgmentally
- reassure and provide information
- encourage appropriate professional help
- foster self-help and other support strategies

Mental Health First Aid USA is administered by the National Center for Community Behavioral Healthcare, the Maryland State Department of Health and Mental Hygiene, and the Missouri Department of Mental Health.

CHAPTER 5

Finding Professional Help

Although you are doing the best you can, at some point you may find that your family member needs the assistance of a mental health professional. This can be a big decision for you and your family. Where to begin? You have so many things to take into consideration and so many choices. You may wonder when the time is right to set this up. Sometimes, it's difficult to know. Any persistent change in your family member's usual baseline self signals that a professional evaluation would be helpful.

Most often it is you, the family members and close friends, who recognize the first signs of depression in someone (Highet, Thompson, and McNair 2005). Family members are often the ones who encourage someone's self-care and early treatment. You may notice small changes well before a physician or therapist who knows him as you do. He most likely respects your opinion and observations. This may help him take the necessary steps to obtain professional help.

You may find it overwhelming when deciding among the many different types of mental health professionals. How do you help your family member pick a provider? What do their different credentials mean? To begin, choosing a mental health provider depends on your family member's needs. As you will learn as you read on, there are different types of providers, each with different skills. Selecting the category of professional is the first step. The next decision depends in part on who is practicing in his local area; their availability; and to a certain extent, your family member's insurance coverage (for example, which providers are in his insurance plan's network and therefore more affordable).

Your family member can also start with his primary care provider (PCP) or family doctor, who will ask him questions about how he is feeling and doing, assess his situation, evaluate his depression, and either begin treatment right away or refer him to a specialist in treating people with mental health problems. It may take a while to diagnose the depression and find a mental health provider with whom he feels comfortable. Some PCPs are experienced in treating early depression, and that may be just what he needs. But more severe types of depression may require a mental health specialist.

You will discover several different types of mental health professionals who are qualified to treat depression. They often work together as a team:

- *Psychiatrists* are medical doctors (MDs) who are specialty trained, licensed, and board certified to treat mental illnesses such as major depression, bipolar disorder, anxiety, and other conditions. They are the mental health providers who evaluate your family member and prescribe medications such as antidepressants.
- *Clinical psychologists* are PhD specialists trained and licensed in evaluating and treating mental illnesses using various kinds of talk therapy, or *psychotherapy*. Psychologists are sometimes referred to as *therapists*. Different types of psychotherapy exist, and each has a different focus and purpose. A psychologist will know which type is suitable for your family member or friend. Talk therapy can help your family member cope with his illness, understand himself better, learn healthy ways to manage stress, make sound life decisions, and adjust to major losses and life transitions. Talk therapy can be done in a one-to-one setting or in small groups of people with similar problems.
- *Licensed clinical social workers* (LICSWs or LCSWs) also provide talk therapy to individuals or in groups.
- In addition, some *nurse practitioners* (NPs), nurses with advanced training, specialize in psychiatric disorders and are

licensed to prescribe antidepressants and other psychiatric medications.

If your family member does not have a PCP or family doctor to refer him to a mental health professional, he can call the patient referral telephone line in the Department of Psychiatry at his local community or university hospital. They can match him with a mental health clinician suited to his symptoms.

The success of your family member's treatment often depends on building a trusting relationship with a therapist or psychiatrist who is a good "fit" for him. The clinician should be someone your family member can speak with freely and get along with. How does your family member find a good psychiatrist or therapist for him personally? Once a referral is made, the best way is usually for him to get the names of several mental health providers and meet with each in person. Encourage him to ask questions of the clinicians he interviews. For example, does the clinician have time to meet with him on a regular basis?

Many people with mood disorders want to know about the provider's training, background, and specific area of interest in psychiatry. Does he or she have experience in treating depression or bipolar disorder? Your family member will want to find out if the clinician is respectful, responsive, and someone he feels comfortable talking to and with whom he can work over time. This may take one or more meetings to figure out. That's okay and expected. Not everyone will be a good match.

Your family member may want to know if the provider has flexible office hours and can accommodate his work or school schedule. He may also be interested in the provider's method of payment and whether his health insurance will cover it. He will want to make sure the mental health clinician will coordinate his care with his PCP. To get the most from his treatment, it is usually recommended that your family member follow all treatment recommendations as prescribed, keep scheduled appointments, arrive to the session sober, be open and honest with the provider, pay attention to the conversation, and do any homework assignments.

If your family member is in crisis and unable to think clearly, is psychotic (loses touch with reality), or is suicidal, his mental health care team will decide on the course of his treatment. This is for his safety. Otherwise, expect that he will be an active participant working with his mental health provider in a collaborative process called *shared decision making*. This means that the provider explains several treatment options to him in a clear and understandable manner. Once that is done to your family member's satisfaction and all of his questions have been answered, then together they decide on the best treatment approach. This process takes into account your family member's preferences and values and respects him as a person. If he encounters a mental health provider who is not willing to share in the decision-making process, he may want to look for another clinician.

While in treatment your loved one may be asked to create a Treatment Contract with his provider, sometimes known as an *Action Plan for Relapse Prevention* (Noonan 2013). This simple document used by some in psychiatry is an agreement that the person who has depression or bipolar disorder creates with his therapist or psychiatrist. It identifies his treatment team, unique triggers and warning signs for worsening mood disorder, the steps to take that have been helpful, the things he will and will not do, and how others can help. It can be quite useful.

Various types of therapy have proven effective for people who have depression. The appropriate kind depends on the person's symptoms and medical history and, to some extent, on the kind of therapy (if any) he has had in the past. Sometimes medication alone is sufficient, sometimes talk therapy alone is sufficient, and sometimes a combination is needed. It can be difficult to predict how anyone will respond to which form of treatment. He may have to try several medications or types of treatment before finding the one that is most effective for his needs. The most effective therapy, in all but the earliest forms of depression, often involves working with both a psychiatrist for medication and a therapist for talk therapy.

One common and effective type of talk therapy is called *Cognitive Behavioral Therapy*, or CBT. This method in psychotherapy is based on the connection between our thoughts, feelings, and actions. CBT teaches a person to identify and change thinking patterns that may be distorted, beliefs that are inaccurate, and behaviors that are unhelpful.

Occasionally, someone who has depression or bipolar disorder is too ill to manage at home or go to outpatient therapy appointments. He may also feel unsafe or suicidal. This situation can overwhelm you as a caretaker. Most people in your position cannot manage this alone.

In this case, your family member needs treatment in the inpatient psychiatry unit of a hospital. Your best first response is to call or encourage him to call his psychiatrist or psychologist, who will arrange a hospital admission. If he has not yet established a mental health provider, your best options are to contact his PCP or take him to your local Emergency Department, where they will evaluate him and make the necessary arrangements.

Once in the hospital, he will be cared for by a treatment team that usually consists of an attending psychiatrist, nurse, and social worker. If he is in a teaching hospital of a university medical center, he will usually have a psychiatry resident and perhaps a medical student attending to him. He may also see a psychologist. The treatment team's role is to see him each day, adjust his medications as required, and encourage him to attend group therapy sessions with other inpatients. Being in the hospital can frighten some people at first, but most leave the hospital feeling better.

A treatment option sometimes offered when medications do not work well or cannot be used for medical reasons is *electroconvulsive therapy* (ECT, also called *shock therapy*). This treatment occurs in the hospital. Your family member or friend receives anesthesia medication to put him to sleep for a few minutes. A very brief, low electric current is sent through small sticky pads, called *electrodes*, which are placed on the scalp. They transmit the current to his brain. It may sound scary, but it does not hurt and he is unaware of the process. Some people may have a mild headache or slight confusion for a few hours afterward. Some people can lose their memory around the time of the treatment. ECT is usually given three times a week for several weeks. A number of people's depression symptoms improve after the first few treatments.

Another treatment proven effective in some people who have depression is *repetitive transcranial magnetic stimulation* (rTMS). This procedure uses a magnetic field to stimulate nerve cells in the brain. rTMS involves placing a special wand called a magnetic coil on a precise location on the scalp. The coil directs magnetic pulses to a portion of the brain involved in mood regulation. Each treatment typically lasts for 40 minutes, 5 times a week for 4 to 6 weeks, then is tapered to twice a week for 3 weeks. The dose and position on the scalp are individualized for each person. rTMS does not require anesthesia, and there is no confusion or memory loss afterward. There may be a mild headache and scalp tingling. Many who have used this treatment have found improvement in their depression symptoms. Various other treatments are currently being studied for their effectiveness.

Often, those receiving treatment for depression find it helpful to speak with others experiencing the same symptoms. Support groups around the country exist just for this purpose. The outpatient psychiatry department at a hospital, or patient (consumer) organizations such as the Depression and Bipolar Support Alliance (DBSA) or the National Alliance on Mental Illness (NAMI), usually sponsor them. The national organizations have local chapters and are open to anyone. These organizations also have sections for friends and family members seeking support for themselves. NAMI conducts a training program for families called Family to Family, which is a 12-week course on accepting and supporting those with mental illness. Approximately 300,000 people have taken it so far and have given excellent feedback.

When Someone Refuses Treatment

Some people have a hard time accepting treatment for depression. Your family member or friend may not believe that treatment will help him, may not recognize the need for treatment, or may just plain refuse to go. If you talk him into going, he may go—but unwillingly.

He might also reject offers of help from anyone. Here are some phrases you may be familiar with: "Get off my back," "Nothing anyone can do will help," and "Nobody understands." Knowing that someone needs treatment but encountering their strong resistance to it can put you in a difficult position.

Unfortunately, you'll find no easy answers or concrete solutions for this one—no magic solutions, clinical trials, or official guidelines from academic societies (except in cases of crisis). There are only suggestions based on families' experiences. Families struggle tremendously trying to convince their loved ones to seek treatment. It is one of the most difficult things people face. Adults have a right to decide for themselves and to refuse treatment, and if they don't perceive the need for it, the conversation becomes one-sided.

Why would someone who desperately needs treatment refuse it? There are several reasons. Your family member or friend may believe that seeking help from a mental health professional means he's a failure. It's hard for someone who has always been able to deal with his own problems to accept help. It may make him feel vulnerable and inadequate. And because of the distorted, negative thinking common in depression, he may perceive any efforts to help as intrusive.

Your family member or friend who has depression may be concerned about the financial burden of receiving treatment. Or his main concern may be privacy issues: he could be afraid that if his friends, coworkers, or employer find out, he'll lose his job, his reputation, or those close to him. He might fear being judged unfairly, criticized, or negatively labeled because of his illness and cut off socially. This is known as the *stigma* of mental illness.

Your family member may also believe that treatment is not effective—at least for him. He may fear becoming dependent on or addicted to medications, dread the side effects they can create, or believe that psychiatric drugs will change who he is. He might also believe the rumors that he will feel like a "zombie" or lose his creativity on medications. Media reports about the adverse effects of medications and negative television advertisements can also contribute to fears about treatment (Sajatovic et al. 2009).

Perhaps your loved one is afraid of the strong emotions that treatment may bring up. This is a common fear in people with mood disorders. Maybe his concerns are based on mistaken beliefs about depression and its treatment.

So what can you do when your family member or friend rejects your help or refuses to go for treatment? Begin by emphasizing that you love him and are concerned about him. Try to calmly explain exactly what you see in him that is different from his usual self. Provide specific examples. You might approach it by saying something like, "You seem to be more down than usual in the past few weeks, and I notice you're not sleeping well. I'm concerned about you. I think this may be a good time for you to speak with Dr. Jones. He can help."

Tell him why you think it's important that he seek help. Mention the symptoms of depression or bipolar disorder he has and point out that treatment may help relieve them. Make him aware that these symptoms and his problems will not improve on their own and that some savvy help may be necessary for him to feel better. Emphasize that you're recommending he get treatment for his own health and well-being. Tell him it may be the only way he can realize his dreams of finishing school, getting back to work, enjoying himself with friends—whatever parts of life he's missing out on. You might mention that having an evaluation doesn't mean he has to decide on or agree to treatment; seeing treatment as an option rather than a foregone conclusion may make him feel more inclined to go. Try to be firm, steady, and persistent.

If misinformation about mood disorders and treatment is behind his reluctance to see a mental health professional, provide him with accurate information about his illness. Once you know his concerns, you or his PCP can address those worries with facts. Gaining information is a powerful tool to counteract resistance. Having knowledge about his illness makes things less scary and may help reverse your family member's resistance to treatment.

He might just feel overwhelmed by the whole idea of going to see a mental health professional. This is where you can help by calling to schedule appointments and arrange health insurance coverage, if required. Search out the names of a few mental health providers in your area and let him decide which he will interview. If he's anxious about going the first few times, offer to go along and sit in the waiting room. You might suggest that he prepare for the appointment by organizing his questions and issues on paper or on a smartphone ahead of time. Do whatever you can to discourage his excuses, remove any obstacles, and make it easier for him to go.

You cannot force a person into treatment unless he is in crisis or, in the rare case, you need to take legal steps to ensure his safety. For example, in the extremely ill, this might mean getting a court order to ensure he takes his medications. While it's difficult to do, respect his right to refuse your help or treatment *unless* you believe he could harm himself or others. Then you must call for professional help or dial 9-1-1 immediately, regardless of his preferences.

Parents or guardians can try to use their influence to get an adolescent into treatment. This may be easier said than done. He can give you a really hard time about not wanting to go. This issue is the cause of many family disruptions. You may have to adopt a tough love approach. Getting him to stay in therapy may be quite another challenge, influenced in part by his relationship with the therapist and the traits of his age group. Try to give your adolescent a sense of personal control by allowing him to make some of the minor decisions about his treatment. This has been an effective strategy in many families. In addition, emphasize that treatment may help him reach some of the goals he's been talking about.

If the person who has depression is a young adult, a spouse, a sibling, or a parent, your options are more limited. You cannot force a child over the age of 18 or other family members to seek treatment. His medical encounters are private, and you have limited access to speak with his health care providers. This is to respect his privacy. Use the strength of your personal connection to him and gentle pressure from other family members to persuade him to seek treatment. A family meeting with his health care provider may finally convince him. Try to focus your comments on your family member's strengths and positive qualities.

There is one thing you can try if he has previously been in treatment and is now experiencing a relapse or recurrence. Encourage him to adopt the terms of a Treatment Contract, or Action Plan for Relapse Prevention, with his mental health provider. This is his plan, described earlier in this chapter, that outlines what to do when the warning signs of worsening mood symptoms occur. You may have some success in getting your family member to abide by his own words in this document and in this way return to treatment.

If your family member with depression is elderly, you may need to focus on his safety. This is particularly true if he lives alone or with an elderly spouse—or seems confused. In some cases he may not remember to take medications as prescribed or may not care. He may not be steady enough to care for himself. The loneliness and chronic medical problems of people in this age group put them at high risk for suicide. When you are not available, another family member or an outside "sitter" may need to be present at all times until the situation improves.

Try not to take your loved one's resistance to therapy—and to your own efforts to help him—personally. You may feel resentful, angry, or frustrated, as these are natural responses to the situation. Use some of the coping strategies outlined in chapter 6 to ease these moments. Take a deep breath, go for a walk, talk to a friend, or get professional help yourself. This can be in individual therapy or by going to a support group for family members. Coping in this situation means paying attention to your feelings, managing your stress, and getting the help *you* need, too.

CHAPTER 6

What You Can Do Now

When you picked up this book, one of your questions might have been, "How do I begin?" As you've read in previous chapters, the first thing to do is to be there, listen, and support your family member or friend who has depression. Self-help and self-care strategies are often useful, and your role is to encourage these efforts. This includes the Basics of Mental Health mentioned in chapter 4 (Noonan 2013). Then try to focus on helping your loved one find professional treatment. After she's engaged in treatment, try to keep the following in mind:

- use active listening, hearing, and empathetic response to communicate
- provide support and hope
- keep realistic expectations for your family member
- help her confront negative thoughts
- encourage her to stick to the Basics of Mental Health
- emphasize that you're in this together—and mean it

It can take several weeks before a person who has depression sees a response to treatment. This is a challenging time. Try to encourage your family member to be patient and stick with the proposed treatment plan.

This chapter provides you with some ideas to help your family member, organized by each of the main symptoms of depression. Keep in mind that she will most often experience a combination of symptoms at the same time. You may then have to overlap and customize your approach to her based on the suggestions below.

Steps for Mood Symptoms

If your family member shows persistent sadness or irritability, your initial response may be to acknowledge this. You can do this by asking open questions and helping her explore her feelings without prying. You could begin with an observation such as, "You seem to be very sad [or irritable] today." Some people open up and begin to talk at this point. If you get no response, you could go on to ask, "What do you think is the reason for this? Has anything happened?" Your family member may realize that her overall sadness is not related to any one thing in particular. Or she may find that something triggered her sadness, such as a major loss or disappointment. It may be one or several things. After identifying the potential cause of her sadness or irritability, you might ask her to think of ways she can deal with it. Is there anything she can do to repair or replace the loss or change the outcome? If so, try to help her find a solution. The following is often an effective strategy in problem solving:

1. Identify the problem.
2. Get accurate information about the problem.
3. Consider the options and alternative solutions.
4. Identify the necessary steps to address the problem.
5. Determine who needs to assist her.

If she finds no concrete ways to change the facts, try to shift the focus of your conversation to coping with it.

Coping strategies are the things we all do to ease the stressors and challenges of daily life. People use an extensive range of tactics for this purpose. They include distraction, relaxation exercises, self-soothing strategies, mindfulness meditation, physical exercise, humor, and other techniques. You might begin by asking your family member what she has done in the past to successfully cope with similar sadness or loss. For example, you could say, "What has helped you in the past when you have felt this way?" If she can identify a strategy or two, which might be something like physical exercise or humor, ask if she's able to engage in those coping mechanisms now. You could say, "Would you like to go for a run now or watch *Ferris Bueller's Day Off?*" This is often a helpful approach for people in similar situations. Examples of other effective coping strategies she might try include:

- Distracting yourself from the problem. Refocus attention on social activities, hobbies, physical exercise, sports, reading, puzzles, music, movies, or volunteering.
- Relaxation techniques. Herbert Benson describes an easy one called *The Relaxation Response* (Benson 2000). Begin by relaxing one muscle group in your body at a time. Slowly relax every other muscle group until all tension is released. Another technique, *mindfulness meditation*, is also easy to fit into your day (Kabat-Zinn 1994). In this practice, you stay present in the moment by paying attention, on purpose and nonjudgmentally, to what you are doing. You let go of worry about the past or future.
- Many people find it helpful to do mindfulness meditation for 5 minutes at a time, once or ideally twice a day. Here's how:
  - Sit in a comfortable chair.
  - Close your eyes.
  - Become aware of your breathing.
  - Focus on each breath.
  - Pay attention to the present moment: your breathing, the sounds around you, and all physical sensations.
  - Observe what you feel, see, and hear without judging it.
  - Continue to focus on each breath, in and out.
  - When intrusive thoughts enter your mind, let them go without judging them or yourself.
  - Return your focus to your breathing.
- Humor. Watch a funny movie or television program or read an amusing book.
- Self-soothing strategies. These involve the five senses—sight (look at something pleasant), taste (prepare and eat good

food), smell (buy fragrant flowers or use a favorite lotion), touch (wear soft, comfortable clothing or get a massage), and hearing (listen to calming music or nature).

- Try to maintain a regular schedule and stay organized. This is a useful strategy for many people with mood disorders. Begin in one or more of the following ways:
  - ° Prioritize what you have to do.
  - ° Break large tasks down into small steps.
  - ° Include pleasurable activities and positive events in your day.
  - ° Keep up with your friends and family.
- Manage life's little daily stressors. Prioritize your day, keep a to-do list, and write things down.

Occasionally, irritability becomes such a strong force that it leads the person who has depression to feel out of control. She may seem argumentative and turn to excesses of work, reckless driving, spending, alcohol or substance abuse, or sexual activity. This pattern is more frequently seen in men and adolescents. If this applies to your family member, it requires your utmost patience. It's a time for you to maintain stability, a steady routine, and structure at home. You may need to set expectations and limits on her behavior and remove any alcohol from the home. You may face resistance. Try to remain calm and firm and don't cave in.

Diminished Interest or Pleasure

Depression may have led your family member to lose interest in her life or things that previously gave her pleasure. They may now seem bland and a waste of time and effort. Work, school, friends, hobbies, sports—why bother? She may prefer to spend time alone, on the sofa watching television, or in her room staring at the wall. Try to engage her in those activities she once enjoyed in small steps and at a pace she can handle now. She doesn't have to actually enjoy the experience; just trying it is enough for now. For example, if she used to like bicycling, you might say, "The weather's great today and I'd really like to get outside. I'd love it if you would join me for a short ride. We could aim for the old lemonade stand." She may or may not respond positively to this approach on any given day.

Try not to set the bar too high. The underlying theory is that "action precedes motivation" (Robert J. McKain, author of *Realize Your Potential*). It means that your family member or friend should not wait to feel interested or motivated before taking action or joining in an activity. Once she begins to do something, the drive to do it will eventually follow and gain momentum. You might ask her to list things she is interested in or used to enjoy. Then try to provide opportunities for her to participate in them. If you provide the opportunity, she may be more likely to engage in the activity. For example, if she likes the family dog, you might ask her to do you a favor and take the dog for a walk. This may help her experience the pleasure of being outside, being with the dog, and helping you. See table 6.1 for some examples of Pleasurable Activities that she might think of doing. Eventually, she may do some of these on her own.

Changes in Appetite or Weight

If your family member or friend has depression, her appetite may change. She may want to eat all the time, hungry or not, or be disinterested in food. This could cause her to eat either too much or too little. This can lead to an unintentional weight gain or loss of five or more pounds over 2 weeks, or more. This adds to depression and a negative body image. She may be eating unhealthy foods, such as fast food or junk food. Poor eating habits can also have an impact on the functioning of her body and brain. Try to promote healthy, balanced meals for your family member and encourage her to follow a healthy eating plan without skipping meals or relying on fast food. Keep unhealthy snacks out of the house and set a good example when at home or eating out. Do it together: make a grocery list, take her food shopping with you, and enlist her help in preparing the meals.

For help with healthy meal preparation, the United States De-

Table 6.1. Pleasurable Activities

Relax (on your own or use a relaxation CD)	Cook
Stretch	Eat a good meal
Get physical exercise	Go on a date
Go for a walk outdoors	Enjoy quiet time
Enjoy the weather	Meditate
Bicycle	Work on a favorite project
Garden	Learn something new
Play a sport	Reach a goal
Watch sports	Travel
Play a game	Work on a favorite hobby
Spend time with friends	Read a good book or magazine
Read the comics	Spend time with family you enjoy
Plan a party	Spend time with children
Go to a party	Volunteer
Give someone a gift	Do a jigsaw puzzle
Watch a good or funny movie	Do Sudoku
Laugh	Do a crossword puzzle
Shop or window shop	Play with a pet
Knit, crochet, or needlepoint	Listen to music
Do woodworking projects	Attend a concert
Enjoy a good fragrance or smell	Play an instrument
Pamper yourself (bubble bath, etc.)	Sing
Get a massage	Learn a new language
Have your hair done	Look at beautiful scenery
Get a manicure or pedicure	Gaze at beautiful art
Visit a museum	And lots of other things . . .

partment of Agriculture (USDA) provides a list of Dietary Guidelines for Americans at www.dietaryguidelines.gov. See table 6.2 for more information.

Difficulty Sleeping

Problems with sleep are common in many people who have depression. She may experience difficulty falling asleep or staying asleep, or she may wake up too early in the morning. She may sleep much longer than usual, with additional naps in the middle of the day, or sleep very little. All of these patterns can be symptoms of depression, and she should speak with her doctor about them. Sleep Hygiene guidelines from the American Academy of Sleep Medicine are listed in table 6.3 (www.sleepeducation.com/essentials-in-sleep/healthy-sleep-habits). This set of guidelines is helpful, and it is important for all of us to follow the guidelines, particularly someone who has a mood disorder.

Physical Restlessness or Slowing Down

Some people who have depression may experience an unusual form of feeling physically restless and agitated, with a constant inner urge to move about and not sit still. This differs from anxiety. Others find they are physically slowed down, which is not the same as fatigue. Some describe it as feeling like an elephant is sitting on them or they are moving through molasses. If your family member or friend finds either of these to be true, she should discuss this with her doctor. A regular physical exercise routine may help.

Fatigue

During an episode of depression, your loved one may feel tired and worn out (Baldwin and Papakostas 2006). Such fatigue can be physical, mental, and emotional. Physical fatigue can include a loss of energy, tiredness, and a reduced ability to exercise. Mental fatigue can involve dulled thinking, problems with focus and attention, or difficulty concentrating. Emotional fatigue frequently involves a lack of motivation, apathy, or weariness. Fatigue can be a symptom of depression, a side effect of medications, or related to insomnia or poor sleep patterns. Make sure your family member or friend discusses the fatigue with her doctor.

If fatigue is a factor in your family member, try to encourage her to stick to the Basics of Mental Health. This means keeping regular sleep hours, with a goal of 7 to 8 hours of sleep per night but not more. Many people with depression find it helpful to follow a healthy and balanced diet, with adequate fluid intake (eight glasses of nonalcoholic fluid per day). Regular physical exercise helps as well. You might become your family member or friend's exercise partner by going out with her for a moderate to fast walk around the block several times per week. This may seem contrary to what you or she may think: How in the world can such a tired person go out and exercise? However, regular exercise is often quite helpful in reversing the symptoms of fatigue. She may be pleasantly surprised at its positive effect.

Feelings of Worthlessness or Guilt

You may find that your family member or friend with depression experiences occasional feelings of worthlessness or guilt without cause. Your best response to her assertions of being "worthless" is to provide active listening and empathic responses. You might begin with asking, "Why do you think you're feeling [worthless, guilty]?" Try to get her to share the reasons that are driving her thoughts. You may find that distorted negative thoughts (see table 4.1) are behind her feelings of worthlessness (Burns 2009). If so, explore what is fact and what may be a distortion in her thinking. You might ask, "I hear you feel you're worthless in life. That must be very painful. Can you tell me more about what makes you feel this way?" Then try to focus on the facts. Remind her of her past successes.

For example, if your friend or family member feels worthless at work, you might say, "I remember last month when you received praise for your part in getting the project done ahead of schedule. How has their opinion of you changed since then?" Your goal is to

Table 6.2. USDA Dietary Guidelines for Americans 2010

Here's a summary list of the key points important to maintaining a healthy body and weight. The USDA Guidelines for 2015 are in process (see www .dietaryguidelines.gov).

» Include a large amount of whole grains, vegetables, and fruits in your diet.

» Eat a variety of vegetables, especially dark green, red, and orange vegetables and beans and peas.

» Replace refined grains with whole grains. At least half of all grains eaten should be whole grains.

» Choose a variety of protein foods, which include seafood, lean meat and poultry, eggs, beans and peas, soy products, and unsalted nuts and seeds. Choose seafood in place of some meat and poultry.

» Use lean, lower calorie proteins instead of high-fat protein.

» Reduce your amount of sugar-sweetened beverages.

» Focus on the total number of calories consumed. Monitor your food intake.

» Be aware of portion size: choose smaller portions or lower-calorie options.

» Eat a nutrient-dense breakfast.

» Reduce daily sodium (salt) intake to less than 2,300 milligrams (mg) per day.

» Get less than 10 percent of calories from saturated fatty acids. Replace them with monounsaturated and polyunsaturated fatty acids.

» Eat fewer than 300 mg per day of dietary cholesterol.

» Increase fat-free or low-fat milk and milk products, such as milk, yogurt, cheese, or fortified soy beverages.

» Use oils to replace solid fats when possible.

» Choose foods that are a rich source of potassium, dietary fiber, calcium, and vitamin D. These include vegetables, fruits, whole grains, and milk and milk products.

» Limit foods that contain synthetic sources of trans fats, such as partially hydrogenated oils.

Source: USDA Dietary Guidelines for Americans, 2010, 7th edition, December 2010.

Table 6.3. Sleep Hygiene

Recommendations to improve your sleep include:

» Keep the same bedtime and wake-up time every day, including weekends. Set an alarm clock if necessary. Get up and out of bed at the same time every morning, even if you've had a bad night's sleep.

» Avoid napping during the day.

» Develop a relaxing ritual before bedtime. Create "downtime" during the last 2 hours before sleep and avoid overstimulation.

» Try going to bed only when you are sleepy.

» Avoid watching the clock or lying in bed frustrated at being unable to fall asleep. Turn the clock away from you.

» If you're unable to fall asleep after 20 to 30 minutes, get out of bed. Relax and distract your mind with a quiet activity in another room (music, reading). Return to bed when you feel sleepy.

» Relaxation exercises before bedtime may help. Examples include progressive muscle relaxation, deep breathing, guided imagery, yoga, or meditation.

» Designate a specific "worry time" earlier in the day or evening to sort out any problems. Writing down reminders for the next day helps to clear your mind before bed.

» Use your bed and bedroom only for sleep, sex, or occasional illness. Eliminate non-sleep activities in bed. Use another room for reading, television, work, or eating.

» Limit the use of caffeine during the day and avoid its use after 12:00 p.m. Note that coffee, tea, colas, chocolate, and some medications contain caffeine.

» Avoid or limit the use of nicotine (tobacco) and alcohol during the day. Don't use them within 4 to 6 hours of bedtime.

» Avoid large meals before bedtime, but don't go to bed hungry. If needed, have a light snack.

» Exercise on a regular basis. Avoid strenuous exercise within 4 to 6 hours of bedtime.

» Create a bedroom environment that favors sound sleep. A comfortable bed in a dark, quiet room is recommended. Minimize light, noise, and hot or cold extremes in room temperature. Room-darkening shades, curtains, earplugs, or a sound machine may be helpful.

» Speak with your doctor if you are having continued difficulty with sleep, including falling asleep, staying asleep, and early or frequent awakenings.

Source: Susan J. Noonan, *Managing Your Depression: What You Can Do to Feel Better* (Johns Hopkins University Press, 2013), 8–9. *Additional References:* American Academy of Sleep Medicine, www.sleepeducation.com/essentials-in-sleep/healthy-sleep-habits, accessed July 16, 2015; www.med.navy.mil/sites/NMCP2/Patient Services/SleepClinicLab/Documents/SleepHygiene.pdf, accessed July 15, 2015.

bring up prior successes that counteract her feelings. The Evidence For and Against exercise in chapter 4 may also be useful.

If your family member or friend feels guilty about something she had little control over, you might ask about the reasons for her feelings and the facts behind them: "What about this situation is making you feel guilty? Do you think you did something to contribute to the outcome?" Find out her level of participation in the event and whether she is carrying the burden for someone else. With no strong facts to back up her feelings of guilt, she is more likely to drop that emotion.

Diminished Ability to Think, Focus, or Concentrate

Trouble concentrating is one of the most common symptoms of depression. It can be particularly frustrating for your family member or friend if she uses her mind every day to perform complex tasks or make major decisions. Focus problems may extend to reading and conversations or recreational activities such as watching a movie or television. It can be annoying and may interfere with her ability to function at her best on a daily basis. Try to help your family member find acceptable work-arounds to compensate. Here are some of the ways you might suggest to help her to meet these challenges:

- Write things down on sticky notes or in a paper or electronic notebook carried daily.
- Use an agenda book to keep track of meetings and appointments.
- Take notes during group and individual meetings and appointments. Ask permission first.
- Break large tasks into small steps and complete them one by one.
- Focus on one thing at a time. Avoid multitasking.
- Read slowly and reread a paragraph as necessary; take notes if needed.
- Watch a short television show rather than a full-length movie for entertainment.

- Learn to say no. A person with depression may need to accept some limitations in what she can realistically do right now. She should be careful in what and how much she takes on. This includes learning to say no to requests for her time when she feels overwhelmed. It may also mean working or going to school on a part-time basis or taking a temporary leave of absence.

Thoughts of Death or Suicide, or a Suicide Plan

Some of those who have depression, including perhaps your family member or friend, may have thoughts of death or suicide. These may be specific, such as wanting to kill herself, or they may come out as a vague statement of not wanting to "be around." She may talk about not wanting to be a burden to others, having no reason to live, or feeling unbearable emotional pain. You may notice a drastic change in her behavior or how she takes care of herself. She may show a loss of interest, withdrawal and isolation from others, changes in sleep or diet, or substance or alcohol use. She may appear depressed, irritable, or anxious. She may have recently experienced a major loss in her life. The Warning Signs of Suicide are presented in table 2.1; Risk Factors for Suicide are presented in table 2.2. The suicidal thoughts may come and go. If you hear any comments like those described, take them very seriously.

If your family member or friend shows any sign of a plan or intent to commit suicide, call for professional help immediately by dialing 9-1-1 or her mental health provider. Suicidal thoughts are a psychiatric emergency. In the meantime, remove anything she might use for this purpose (pills or weapons, for example) and do not leave her alone.

CHAPTER 7

Anticipating Recovery—
Skills to Have in Place

Perhaps you have heard the saying "Build your life raft before you need it." You might wonder what it has to do with mood disorders, particularly with your family member or friend who has depression. *Life raft* refers to the coping and adaptive skills people have successfully used to manage depression. Here, it means you encourage your family member or friend to learn these skills when he feels well so they are available to him when depression strikes.

Why is this important? Those who cope effectively with the negative effects of stress and their illness may "bounce back" more readily after an episode of depression or bipolar disorder (Catalano et al. 2011; Wingo et al. 2010). This is known as *resilience*, defined in the online brochure "The Road to Resilience" by the American Psychological Association (APA) (www.apa.org/helpcenter/road-resilience.aspx) as the "process of adapting well in the face of adversity, trauma, threats, and significant sources of stress—such as family and relationship problems, serious health problems, or workplace and financial stress."

Think of resilience as an ongoing process of dealing with the difficult times in our lives, facing challenges (such as an illness like depression or bipolar disorder), finding solutions, and recovering from setbacks. Having resilience means that your loved one learns effective ways of thinking and responding during difficult situations. Resilience involves having adaptive behaviors and coping skills such as problem solving, managing stress, facing one's fears, mastering challenges, regulating one's emotions, and learning the consequences of one's behaviors. These coping strategies can help a person survive and thrive despite hardship.

Resilience includes hope for recovery and a sense of determination. Adapting to stress and difficult life events is a complicated process. We learn some of it from our parents and family. It is also likely that genetic factors influence our resilience to adversity (Stein, Campbell-Sills, and Gelernter 2009). On the other hand, resilience doesn't require a person to have exceptional or unique traits. Rather, it comes from the common inner qualities that surface when humans adapt to stress (APA Road to Resilience 2015; Masten 2001).

You might wonder what makes some people more resilient than others. Southwick and Charney (2012) looked at this very question. They surveyed three groups of people who had experienced extraordinary adversity in life and survived remarkably well. In the survey responses, they found ten personal characteristics or coping strategies common to those in each of these three groups. They found that people who have resilience used many of these strategies, which they call *Resilience Factors*. They are presented for you here in table 7.1.

"The Road to Resilience" identifies the following additional characteristics important to developing resilience:

- Avoid seeing crises as insurmountable. Develop confidence in your ability to solve problems.
- Accept change as a part of living.
- Make realistic plans and move toward them.
- Take decisive action in difficult situations.
- Nurture a positive view of yourself. Trust your own instincts.
- Keep things in perspective.
- Maintain flexibility and balance in life.

The APA also notes that caring and supportive relationships, in and outside the family, are essential to building resilience. They create love and trust, provide role models, and offer encouragement. Note the common points and crossover in these two lists of resilience characteristics.

People use various strategies to learn resilience skills. They depend on the individual; the resources he has available through family and friends; and the characteristics of his culture, religion, and community. The culture or community a person was raised in might influence whether and how much he connects with others, communicates his feelings, or deals with adversity. Some people are very private and uncomfortable sharing their feelings, while others reveal every last detail of their emotional life.

What does all of this mean, and how does it apply to your family member or friend? Using the Resilience Factors, here are some ways you can help him build resilience. The hope is that these skills will lend him a greater ability to face the challenges of his illness and recover more readily when mood fluctuations occur. He may also be better able to manage stress and feelings of anxiety (APA Resilience Guide 2015).

Table 7.1. Resilience Factors

1. Maintain an optimistic but realistic outlook.
2. Confront your fears.
3. Rely on your inner-core values and altruism.
4. Draw on religious or spiritual practices.
5. Seek and accept social support.
6. Imitate resilient role models.
7. Attend to your physical, mental, and emotional health and well-being.
8. Challenge your mind to maintain brain fitness.
9. Try to maintain cognitive and emotional flexibility—accept that which you cannot change and focus on what you can change.
10. Look for meaning, purpose, and opportunity in the face of adversity.

Source: S. M. Southwick and D. S. Charney, *Resilience: The Science of Mastering Life's Greatest Challenges* (Cambridge University Press, 2012).

How to Help Your Loved One Build Resilience

There are a lot of strategies here. Don't think that you have to master all of them. Instead, choose one or two you feel may work for your family member and give them a try. If they don't work or they are too hard for you, choose another one or two. Try to

- provide unconditional, nonjudgmental love and support. It's important to support your family member or friend as he works to build resilience.
- maintain an optimistic but realistic outlook for your family member or friend with depression. This means holding a reasonable view of the future that involves hope and the confidence that things will turn out well, with enough hard work. Then help your family member or friend embrace this realistic attitude about his future. Help him avoid unattainable dreams as goals. Focus on what he can do now with effort and encouragement. It may be difficult, but try to remain hopeful about his future. No one can predict the course of anyone's depression or recovery. Encourage him to continue with his chosen path in life, even if at a slower pace for now. Sometimes, one's life plans have to be put on hold for a little while during an illness. Consider it a temporary pause and not the final stop.
- keep an optimistic attitude when your family member or friend's moods fluctuate. You may find this very hard to do. Try the following:
  - Remind him that this situation won't last forever.
  - Help him keep the illness or negative event in perspective. Remind him that although depression is a biological illness that's a part of his life, it does not *define* him.
  - Confront his negative thoughts and emotions using the method from chapter 4. Encourage him to recall past achievements to find evidence for the positive and evidence against his negative views of himself and the world.

Urge him to seek an outside opinion of himself from those he respects. Positive thinking (including hopefulness and a positive view of himself and the world) and positive life events can act as a buffer against depression symptoms in vulnerable people (Haeffel and Vargas 2011; Mak, Ng, and Wong 2011).

    ○ Have your family member or friend recall the inner strengths and resources he has used to deal with past problems. Encourage him to use them now. For example, his perseverance or sense of humor might help him through a difficult time.

    ○ Bring up past successes that obviously show his strengths and abilities. Then offer him new opportunities to demonstrate those strengths and reinforce his confidence.

- guide your family member or friend toward concrete and realistic goals. Urge him to plan his future in small, incremental steps. Encourage him to gain the skills to reach his goal, gather the support he needs, and take the action to succeed.

- be supportive as your family member or friend learns to face his fears. Fear can interfere with moving forward and recovering from depression. It may be helpful if he first accepts his fears, gathers information about them, and then makes plans to confront them. Many people find this far better than passively wishing them away.

- help him guide his life by the core values he has learned over time and the benefits he has received from reaching out to help others. *Core values* are the principles, such as honesty, respect, fairness, and compassion, by which we lead our lives. Remind him to rely on his inner sense of right and wrong (his *moral compass*) during periods of stress. Suggest he practice altruism, the act of helping others. Volunteering can bring great benefits as he works to build resilience.

- consider whether a spiritual or religious approach is useful. Southwick and Charney (2012) found that some people turn to religion or spirituality to cope with adversity. This approach, they discovered, can lead to lower levels of depression and restore hope and a more balanced view.

- increase your family member or friend's social support network. This is a foundation upon which to build resilience. Close relationships build strength and may protect him during stressful times. Isolation and decreased social support frequently lead to increased stress and depression (Vanderhorst and McLaren 2005).

- use role modeling as a tool to increase resilience as described below. Family members and caregivers often play the role model who demonstrates skills and behaviors your family member or friend may imitate. Role models help build resilience through their words and actions. Role models can help guide a person as he learns to manage stress; handle disappointment, difficult life situations, and relationships; make major decisions; and care for himself physically and emotionally. You might try the following techniques (Southwick and Charney 2012):

  ○ Provide consistent and reliable support.
  ○ Inspire and motivate him by your actions.
  ○ Foster self-esteem.
  ○ Model right versus wrong.
  ○ Show how to handle difficult situations.
  ○ Model how to control impulses.
  ○ Advise how to delay gratification and soothe oneself.
  ○ Demonstrate how to take responsibility for oneself and one's own actions.

- encourage your family member or friend to take care of his physical and cognitive self (his mind) and learn self-care. Following a daily physical exercise program is important. Regular exercise acts as an aid to depression treatment and lends a sense of self-confidence and self-respect (Dunn et al. 2005; Mead et al. 2009). Physical training helps to improve mood, thinking, self-confidence, and emotional resilience. It also improves mental and emotional health and well-being and decreases the symptoms of depression (Rethorst and Trivedi 2013; Trivedi et al. 2006). In addition to physical exercise, daily brain activity keeps the mind sharp and ready to face life's challenges. Encourage your family member or friend to read, do puzzles, or play challenging mind games rather than sit aimlessly on the couch in front of the television.

- help your family member or friend accept what he cannot change and focus on what he can do now. Remind him that change is a part of living. Certain goals may no longer be attainable as a result of his illness.

- support your family member or friend as he learns to control and tolerate his strong feelings, emotions, and impulses. This is frequently done with a therapist, but a family member can reinforce it at home.

- encourage your family member or friend to seek a purpose in life rather than aimlessly wandering from one school or job to the next. How do you do this? Help him find something he enjoys and does well. Support him in completing its required educational or training program. This could involve school, work, family, sports, social service, or volunteer activities.

- help him identify and build on the strengths and personal qualities he already has. Sometimes depression makes it difficult for a person to see them in himself. Try using the strategies outlined in chapter 4.

- work with your family member or friend as he develops new problem-solving skills. Reinforce those he already has. See chapter 6 for an outline of ideas to encourage problem solving.

If your family member or friend is temporarily unable to think clearly or experiences depression, hopelessness, and lack of energy, he may find it hard to learn the new skills needed to build resilience (Southwick and Charney 2012). But although his overwhelming thought processes are often negative, his self-confidence may diminish, and his ability to manage strong feelings frequently wanes, these skills aren't impossible to learn. It often just takes the right timing and perseverance on his part.

CHAPTER 8

Caring for the Caregivers

After attempting many of the things mentioned in this book to help your family member or friend who has depression or bipolar disorder, you may feel emotionally and physically exhausted. You may also find that her illness personally affects you in other ways. Perhaps you fear that you may have done something to cause your family member's unhappiness. In addition, the interactions you have with her may be difficult and stressful for several reasons. Those with depression often have trouble reciprocating in a relationship. If that's the case, you may find it challenging to keep giving of yourself when you are receiving little in return. For example, you may offer love but feel it's not returned, you may offer sympathy but be told "you don't understand," or you may offer support but be told it's not enough or not the "right kind." This can make you feel guilty, then angry, then guilty for feeling angry.

Caregivers sometimes become frustrated with their family member or friend for her behavior and mood swings. You may feel ready to abruptly say, "Snap out of it!" You may wonder why your mother or spouse or daughter puts you through an emotional roller coaster by being inconsistently irritable or stopping medications. This can lead to anger and may destroy relationships.

You may eventually start feeling bad about yourself. You may feel sad, begin to doubt your abilities, or feel helpless at being unable to solve your family member's problems. Some caregivers develop depression, related to the caregiving or not (if you are concerned that you have depression, see the last part of this chapter). You may come to resent your friend or family member and then grow angry toward her. Or maybe you desire to escape the situation entirely. This can make you think you are selfish and unloving, which is certainly not true. If you find yourself in a difficult situation with your loved one, you may need to take a break from the moment. Take a breather by going outside for a walk or doing something to care for yourself.

Illness in a family member may influence you and your family's day-to-day routine, social activities, opportunities, finances, and personal relationships. Taking care of someone who has depression can be a full-time job. Everything seems to stop to accommodate her emotional issues and scheduled appointments. Perhaps the time you spend enjoying your own friends and other relatives has been put on hold because your family member's illness takes priority. You may even lose friends if they are unable to understand depression as a biologically based illness. Many families experience a financial strain due to loss of income. Your ill family member may have stopped working. Caring for her may have forced you to cut back your own work hours. This is on top of her medical expenses.

If your family member who has depression is a spouse or partner, other factors may affect your relationship. You may start assuming different roles, with the healthy person taking on more responsibility for the household duties, family, and relationship. Your daily routine and social life may change. You could have intimacy and sexual difficulties as well. This can result from the depression and some of the medications used to treat it. If your marriage or relationship had troubles before your loved one's illness, they may continue or grow worse now. Take this opportunity to openly communicate with your partner and have her speak with her provider about the problem.

You, as the healthy one, may feel a loss and sense of isolation since your depressed loved one is not as available to you as in the past. If neither of you recognize that she is experiencing clinical depression, you may wonder why she's behaving so negatively, is withdrawn, or is irritable. In addition, a depressed person's fatigue, hopelessness, constant worry, and lack of interest can be disruptive to the stability of a family. Understanding that depression may be an issue will help you and your partner better prepare for these problems.

When a partner or other family member is being treated for a mood disorder, it can be very difficult to be left out of the loop on such an important matter that affects the whole family. You can try to get her to talk about issues that impact you and the family, using a respectful and gentle approach. Help her to realize that you are in this together. Try to understand that she may have times when she does not want to open up to you. Also, don't expect her to share the details of deeply private therapy conversations.

A parent's or sibling's mental illness frequently affects the children in the family. This is true even if it's not spoken of openly in the home. Children usually observe the behavior and language of their parents and pick up on the subtle cues of depression. A child may also be at risk for developing depression later in life when raised in a family in which one parent has the illness (Barker et al. 2012; Batten et al. 2012; Pilowsky et al. 2006; Weissman et al. 2004; Weissman et al. 2015). Try to be open and honest with children in an age-appropriate way. Explain what's going on before their imaginations take over.

For example, if you have a young child you might say, "Daddy's not feeling very well right now. He is very sad and has trouble doing some of the things he usually likes to do. We all have to be very patient now. He talked with his doctor and is getting medication so that he will feel better. He's going to be okay. He still loves you very much." The siblings of someone who has depression may need the same type of attention.

The vulnerability of a depressed person and the stability of the family are often connected. If the family has serious issues or family members have medical or mental illnesses themselves, depression in their loved one is likely to worsen or take longer to resolve (DePaulo and Horvitz 2002). In addition, families often vary in their ability to adapt to stress. Some families cope well; some, not so well. Their social and financial resources, the family makeup, the availability of social support, and the presence of other illnesses may influence this. The family's inability to adequately respond to stress may prolong a person's depression episode (DePaulo and Horvitz 2002).

Dealing with a mood disorder in a family member is a lot to handle. It requires patience, persistence, determination, and courage on your part. Try to be objective. Do your best to avoid getting caught up in the whirlwind of what your family member is saying and doing. Try to focus on her underlying feelings and emotional pain and respond to those. All of this can put pressure on you and other family members. It can lead to burnout unless you take steps to monitor and care for yourselves.

What exactly is burnout? *Burnout* refers to the symptoms and emotions you may have from the stress of caring for someone. It's a kind of fatigue; the sense of having reached the limits of your endurance and your ability to cope (Golant and Golant 2007). Burnout is the result of too many demands on your strength, resources, time, and energy. The situation goes beyond your ability to deal with it. Burnout is a fairly common experience among caregivers. When experiencing burnout, you may feel a combination of physical and emotional factors, such as:

- Headaches
- Difficulty sleeping (insomnia)
- Lack of energy
- Muscle aches
- Stomach upsets
- Frustration, irritability, or anger
- Sadness
- Pessimism
- Resentfulness
- Disinterest and apathy
- Depression

How do you protect against burnout and keep from losing yourself in your family member's illness? The best way is to take time to care for yourself. Paying attention to your own needs does not mean you are ignoring your loved one's needs (Rosen and Amador 1996). Instead, it enables you to be a more available and productive support person.

Do your best to care for yourself physically, mentally, and emotionally. Try to get sufficient and regular sleep, exercise, and relaxation. Many caregivers find balance and relaxation in a yoga class or meditation exercises. Next, follow a balanced diet and nutrition plan as outlined in table 6.2. Try to keep up with your own friends and support people and see them regularly—don't brush them aside for your caregiver role. Some people find brief supportive psychotherapy helpful at these times. This might include joining a support group specifically for friends and families of those with depression. In addition, do your best to keep your usual routine and structure in your life.

Try to manage life's little daily stressors before they explode into unmanageable problems. You might break large tasks into smaller projects, prioritize the demands placed on you, and learn to say no on occasion. Look to your own needs and wants, doing what increases your own self-esteem and pleasure (hobbies, interests, skills, or volunteer work). Treat yourself to something special every once in a while—a meal out, a bouquet of flowers, a massage—and don't feel guilty doing so. Many people find it refreshing to take time for the Pleasurable Activities listed in table 6.1.

Rosen and Amador (1996) provide guidelines to help you care for yourself while in a support role, including:

- Learn all you can about the illness. The more you learn, the better you will be able to cope with it. A clear understanding may empower you to help your family member even more. Be an informed consumer: learn the facts, check the provider's credentials, and weigh the evidence on suggested treatment options.

- Have realistic expectations of how you can help. Set clear limits on what you can do and try not to overcommit. Make sure your family member understands this.
- Give unconditional support to your family member with depression.
- Aim for a regular routine in your own life. Work, eat, sleep, exercise, socialize, and relax. Keep those a priority, and try not to allow your family member's needs to overshadow them.
- If you can, share your feelings about your life with your family member. Your ability to open up may go far in connecting with her.
- Don't take anything your family member says personally. Remember that she is seeing the world through a negative, distorted lens. Depression can impair her ability to express her thoughts, wishes, and needs. Try to understand that she may believe she is unlovable and unworthy of affection.
- Many caregivers find it useful to seek help from friends and other family members. This might include picking up the laundry, walking the dog, going to the post office, or taking the time to listen and support you. You cannot do this alone.
- Work together as a team with your family member. Avoid becoming a controlling force in her life.

Many people find success with the strategies learned in this chapter. Don't expect to master it all at once—pick one tactic at a time and work on that until you feel comfortable, then move on to another if you choose.

But what if you have tried to do many of these things and find yourself feeling sad, down, or thinking that you, too, may be depressed? That is not common, but it can happen. First, try to follow the Basics of Mental Health (Noonan 2013) outlined in chapter 4. Aim for balance and a familiar routine in your life. Engage as much support for yourself as possible from your close friends and other family members. This may also be the time for you to speak with your primary care provider or family doctor, who will ask you questions and assess your situation. You and he or she can then decide if you need to see a mental health professional in the short term. Many people find a support group for family members like you to be particularly helpful as well.

CHAPTER 9

Dos and Don'ts

We each have our way of coping with stressful situations and an illness like depression or bipolar disorder. Personal experiences from our past flavor the illness, our relationships, our life events, and our work. As a result, we all have varying needs when it comes to receiving help from others. For some of us, receiving such help is a major challenge. It may make us feel vulnerable, needy, inadequate, or dependent. Others accept help much more easily. Try to remember this when you offer to help someone who has depression.

This chapter appears quite simple at first glance, but don't be fooled—a lot of key material is presented here. It can be a most useful reference or tool in your efforts to aid someone in distress. Some find it helpful to review each key point thoughtfully and slowly.

DO TRY TO:

- Be present and give your family member or friend your full attention.
- Provide unconditional love and support.
- Listen.
- Do what you say you are going to do.
- Maintain hope and a realistic optimism.
- Let him know you care.
- Validate his feelings and make him feel worthwhile.
- Know the symptoms of depression and mania.
- Watch for the warning signs of worsening depression or mania and know when to encourage professional help.

- Be a positive role model.
- Remind him of his special qualities (such as a sense of humor).
- Call his attention to similar challenges he has successfully met.
- Encourage him to face his fears.
- Urge him to strive to achieve his goals.
- Respect his choice about how much he wants to share. Some people are very private about their feelings. Others may want to talk about their depression. If someone confides in you, keep the conversation to yourself. Ask him how much he wants others to know.
- Discuss treatment decisions with him if asked, but don't offer advice. Respect his decisions even if you disagree.
- Offer to help with routine tasks, but don't take over. Look for ways to facilitate his self-care.
- Help in concrete, specific ways (such as picking up groceries, walking the dog, or going with him to an appointment).
- Include him in daily activities or social events. Let him be the one to determine if it's too much to manage.
- Keep your relationship as normal and balanced as possible. He may appreciate conversations and activities that don't involve depression.
- Expect him to have good days and bad days, emotionally and physically.
- Remember that greater patience and compassion may be necessary at times.
- Respect your own limits.
- Take care of yourself. You won't be effective at helping another if you are burned out.
- Be aware of the Warning Signs of Suicide. Call 9-1-1 if you are concerned.

TRY NOT TO:

- Offer advice or judge your family member or friend.
- Compare his experience to your own or others.
- Blurt out reassuring words automatically when he expresses despair. This can cause him to feel dismissed rather than supported. Before just saying, "You'll be fine," think about whether you're only trying to calm your own anxiety.
- Take things too personally. It's common for him to sometimes be more quiet or irritable than usual.
- Be afraid to talk about depression or mania.
- Fear asking him about suicidal thoughts, plans, or attempts.
- Blame him for his illness, thoughts, or feelings. Understand that this is a biologically based illness.
- Use cliché's and quick responses, such as "Snap out of it!"
- Promise anything you cannot deliver.

For additional recommendations, see A. Yeung, G. Feldman, M. Fava, *Self-Management of Depression: A Manual for Mental Health and Primary Care Professionals* (Cambridge University Press, 2010), appendix C.

Conclusion

Thank you for taking this journey with me. In the process I hope that you've gained understanding and learned new skills. I hope that knowing what to say and do for your family member or friend who has depression or bipolar disorder makes things better for you both.

I started by reviewing the basics of major depression and bipolar disorder and defining the symptoms. Most caregivers find this background information helps them better understand what they're dealing with. Now you also have a better idea of how depression may differ in adults, adolescents, men, and women.

I discussed how anxiety symptoms may affect those with depression as well. You now have a sense of what to look for if you suspect your family member or friend has a mood disorder. You'll be alert for changes from his usual self in general appearance, actions, thoughts (including suicide), and feelings.

Next, I hope you learned communication and support skills to use daily when interacting with your family member or friend. These include active listening, using open body language, and asking open-ended questions. One of the most effective skills to practice is the empathic response, showing you recognize and understand the emotions she's feeling and where they come from.

Along the way I gave you some strategies to use every day. For example, the chapter on Helpful Approaches outlines why and how to treat her normally, provide hope, have realistic expectations, help her confront her negative thoughts, and be aware of her warning signs. It goes on to list the Basics of Mental Health for use in everyday life. Other important approaches you may find helpful include setting boundaries and learning about a program called Mental Health First Aid.

Once you're ready to use these skills, you may need to know when to call for professional help. Chapter 5, which reviewed the different types of mental health providers and treatments available, can help. Armed with that information, you'll be better able to assist with finding the most effective level of care needed. You also now have a sense of how to respond if your family member refuses help or professional treatment.

Once you became familiar with depression symptoms and the communication and support skills to use, I presented a detailed approach, based on each symptom, to help your family member. Understand that someone with depression may experience several symptoms at a time. Your approach to them will overlap.

Next, I shared with you the concept of resilience—a person's ability to bounce back after a difficult time. When you foster resilience in your friend or family member who has depression, she is more likely to hardily weather the storms of depression and bipolar disorder. You as a role model can encourage her and teach her resilience skills.

Finally, I stressed the importance of taking care of yourself. Caring for a family member or a close friend with any medical problem, particularly mood disorders, is both stressful and time consuming. You can't help her if your energy and resources are spent or if you resent her illness. Take the time to get enough sleep, eat a balanced diet, get regular exercise, manage your stress, keep up with your own social contacts and activities, and pursue the hobbies that sustain you. Make sure you have pleasurable experiences in your day. This may help you avoid burnout. Your family member or friend will thank you for this.

This book contains a lot of material. Don't expect to master it right away or after one reading. It takes time, practice, and patience to work on any new skill. I recommend you choose one or two approaches you think may be effective and work on each one slowly.

Focus on one section of a chapter at a time. Read it as many times as needed. Once you feel comfortable using a skill, you may want to learn a new one. You and the person you are helping will likely notice the difference—and feel better for it.

Good luck!

Glossary

Active listening • a way to communicate that signals to a person that you are fully present and paying attention to what he is saying.

Automatic negative thoughts • thoughts that occur quickly and involuntarily during episodes of depression and cause distress. They arise because (1) negative events dominate the thinking of someone who has depression, and (2) the depressed mind tends to interpret and twist things in a negative direction. These thoughts don't accurately reflect reality.

Bipolar depression • a biologically based illness that negatively affects one's thoughts, emotions, and behaviors. It is relapsing and remitting yet treatable and alternates with episodes of extreme elevated mood (mania or hypomania). It affects relationships, activities, interests, and many other aspects of life. Bipolar depression is thought to involve a dysfunction of the network of *neurons* (brain cells) in the brain.

Bipolar disorder • a chronic mood disorder that has a major impact on daily life. Also known as *manic-depressive disorder*, it is thought to result from a dysfunction of the network of neurons in the brain. Bipolar disorder is characterized by episodes of extreme elevated mood or irritability (mania or hypomania) followed by episodes of depression.

Cognitive Behavioral Therapy (CBT) • a kind of talk therapy, or *psychotherapy*, that addresses the connection between our thoughts, feelings, and actions. CBT teaches a person to identify and change thinking patterns that may be distorted, beliefs that are inaccurate, and behaviors that are unhelpful.

Cognitive distortions • errors in thinking that twist a person's interpretation of an event. This is common in depression. CBT uses exercises to challenge and replace the negative and distorted thoughts with more realistic thoughts.

Coping strategies • the things we do to ease the stressors and challenges of daily life. Coping includes problem solving, self-soothing, relaxation, distraction, humor, mindfulness meditation, and other techniques.

Depression • a biologically based illness that negatively affects one's thoughts, emotions, and behaviors. Depression is a relapsing and remitting yet treatable illness of the mind and body. It affects relationships, activities, interests, and many other aspects of life. Depression is thought to involve a dysfunction of the network of neurons in the brain. This may happen when certain life experiences occur in a susceptible person.

Distorted thinking • errors in thinking that twist someone's interpretation of an event. CBT uses a series of exercises to challenge and replace the negative and distorted thoughts that accompany depression.

Empathic response • a response that tries to identify with and understand someone's feelings or problems as if they were our own. We respond in a way that shows we recognize and understand what she is feeling and where it came from.

Hypomania • an elevated, hyper mood that is part of bipolar disorder. It comes in episodes that alternate with bipolar depression, and the pattern is unique to each person. The symptoms are similar to mania. Hypomania is of shorter duration and less intense than mania.

Major depression • a treatable, biologically based illness that negatively affects one's thoughts, feelings, and behaviors. Depression is a relapsing and remitting illness of the mind and body. It affects relationships, activities, interests, and various other aspects of life. Depression is thought to involve a dysfunction of the network of neurons in the brain. This may happen when certain life experiences occur in a susceptible person.

Mania • an elevated, hyper mood that is part of bipolar disorder. It comes in episodes unique to each person and alternates with bipolar depression. The symptoms of elevated mood affect our thoughts, feelings, and behaviors. They include an inflated sense of self, increased physical energy, a decreased need for sleep, racing thoughts, irritability, high-risk behaviors, and others.

Mental Health First Aid • a training program that teaches skills to help a person who has a mental health problem or is in a mental health crisis. It is given until appropriate professional treatment is received or the crisis resolves.

Mood disorders • conditions of the brain that involve the state of mind—the part of our inner self that colors and drives thoughts, feelings, and behaviors. Mood disorders are treatable biological illnesses. Mood disorders include major depression and bipolar disorder.

Realistic optimism • a reasonable view of the future that involves hope and the confidence that things will turn out well, with enough hard work and determination.

Resilience • the ability to face challenges (such as an illness like depression or bipolar disorder), find solutions, and recover from setbacks.

Resilience factors • a set of characteristics common to those who adapt well to stressful times.

Rumination • when a person repeatedly thinks about the same thing.

Sleep hygiene • the personal habits, behaviors, and environmental conditions that affect a person's sleep. These include going to bed and waking up at the same time 7 days a week, reserving the bed for sleep only, avoiding caffeine after noon, and more. These habits have a positive impact on the quality and quantity of sleep.

Risk Factors for Suicide • a set of personal life history items that may make it more likely that a person will take her life.

Warning Signs of Suicide • a set of behaviors that may indicate a person is contemplating harming himself or taking his life.

Support • the time spent listening, hearing, and acknowledging the emotions that someone is experiencing. It also includes advocating on his behalf.

Triggers • events or circumstances that may cause someone distress and lead to an increase in symptoms of depression.

Warning signs of depression • distinct changes from a person's usual thoughts, feelings, behaviors, routine, or self-care noticed by others. These changes may indicate a new or worsening episode of depression.

Resources

Some of the Many Books That May Be of Interest

Herbert Benson. *The Relaxation Response*. Avon; 1975, revised 2000.

David B. Burns. *Feeling Good: The New Mood Therapy*. HarperCollins; 2009.

Nell Casey. *Unholy Ghost: Writers on Depression*. William Morrow; 2001.

Roger Fisher and William Ury. *Getting to Yes: Negotiating Agreement without Giving In*. Penguin; 1983, 1991, 2012.

Kay Redfield Jameson. *An Unquiet Mind: A Memoir of Mood and Madness*. Vintage Books (Random House); 1995.

Jon Kabat-Zinn. *Wherever You Go, There You Are: Mindfulness Meditation in Everyday Life*. Hyperion; 1994.

David J. Miklowitz. *The Bipolar Disorder Survival Guide: What You and Your Family Need to Know*. Guilford Press; 2010.

Francis Mark Mondimore. *Bipolar Disorder: A Guide for Patients and Families*. 2nd ed. Johns Hopkins University Press; 2006.

Francis Mark Mondimore. *Depression, the Mood Disease*. 3rd ed. Johns Hopkins University Press; 2006.

Francis Mark Mondimore and Patrick Kelly. *Adolescent Depression: A Guide for Parents*. 2nd ed. Johns Hopkins University Press; 2015.

Susan J. Noonan. *Managing Your Depression: What You Can Do to Feel Better*. Johns Hopkins University Press; 2013.

Deborah Sichel and Jeanne Watson Driscoll. *Women's Moods: What Every Woman Must Know about Hormones, the Brain, and Emotional Health*. Quill; 1999.

Andrew Solomon. *The Noonday Demon: An Atlas of Depression*. Scribners; 2001.

William Styron. *Darkness Visible*. Vintage Books; 1990.

William Ury. *Getting Past No: Negotiating in Difficult Situations*. Bantam; 1993, 2007.

Mark Williams, John Teasdale, Zindel Segal, and Jon Kabat-Zinn. *The Mindful Way through Depression: Freeing Yourself from Chronic Unhappiness*. Guilford Press; 2007.

Organizations That May Be of Interest

Depression and Bipolar Support Alliance (DBSA), www.dbsalliance.org

The DBSA's mission is to provide "hope, help, support, and education to improve the lives of people who have mood disorders." The DBSA has local chapters with support groups that meet regularly, national educational meetings, online wellness tools, an advocacy center, and training programs for peer specialists. You can share ideas in its online community, the Facing Us Clubhouse.

National Alliance for Mental Illness (NAMI), www.nami.org

NAMI is the largest grassroots mental health organization in the United States. It provides information about mental illness, treatment options, support groups, and programs. You can go online to find a link to your local NAMI chapter. NAMI runs a highly regarded training program called Family to Family, a 12-week evidence-based course on accepting and supporting those with mental illness. Approximately 300,000 people have completed it.

American Foundation for Suicide Prevention (AFSP), www.afsp.org

The AFSP funds research, provides educational programs for professionals, and educates the public about mood disorders and suicide prevention. It also promotes policies and legislation on suicide prevention and provides resources for survivors of suicide loss and people at risk.

Beyond Blue, www.beyondblue.org
This Web site of the National Depression Initiative of Australia contains information for those with depression and anxiety.

National Institute of Mental Health (NIMH), www.nimh.nih.gov
This national organization supports research on mental illness and provides information about depression and bipolar disorder, including current research and clinical trials.

Online Information That May Be of Interest

American Psychological Association (APA), The Road to Resilience, http://www.apa.org/helpcenter/road-resilience.aspx
This online brochure defines *resilience* as the "process of adapting well in the face of adversity, trauma, threats, and significant sources of stress—such as family and relationship problems, serious health problems, or workplace and financial stress." It provides personal strategies for developing and enhancing resilience.

Women's Mental Health, www.womensmentalhealth.org
This online library of articles, a blog, and newsletters sponsored by the Department of Psychiatry of the Massachusetts General Hospital (MGH) provides the latest information on mental health for women in all stages of life. The focus is primarily on mood disorders during the reproductive (childbearing) and menopausal years. There are also links to both the Clinical Program and the Research Program at the MGH Center for Women's Mental Health.

Physical Activity Tracker, www.choosemyplate.gov/SuperTracker/physicalactivitytracker.aspx
This interactive online tool makes it simple to pick the type of physical exercise you enjoy and track how many times and for how long you do it each day and week. You can also record the intensity of your exercise session and set a weekly target goal. Additionally, this tool allows you to see your daily calorie limit and daily food group targets. It's an easy way to stay motivated and follow your progress.

Physical Activity Guidelines, www.cdc.gov/physicalactivity, www.health.gov/PAGuidelines

This online site contains guidelines on how much exercise you need at every age, how to add physical activity to your life, and how to measure the intensity of your physical exercise session.

United States Department of Agriculture (USDA)
Dietary Guidelines for Americans 2010, www.health.gov/ dietaryguidelines, www.choosemyplate.gov

This is the United States site for diet and nutritional guidance for all Americans. It includes information on nutrients and their health benefits, portion sizes, weight management and calories, daily food plans, nutrition during pregnancy, and physical activity, as well as interactive tools.

References

Preface

Wingo AP, Wrenn G, Pelletier T, et al. Moderating effects of resilience on depression in individuals with a history of childhood abuse or trauma exposure. *J Affect Disord.* 2010;126(30):411–414.

Introduction

American Foundation for Suicide Prevention (AFSP). www.afsp.org/understanding-suicide/facts-and-figures. Accessed July 2015.

American Psychiatric Association (APA). *Diagnostic and Statistical Manual of Mental Disorders (DSM-5).* 5th ed. American Psychiatric Association; 2013.

Martin LA, Neighbors HW, Griffith DM. The experience of symptoms of depression in men vs women: Analysis of the National Comorbidity Survey replication. *JAMA Psychiatry.* 2013;70(10):1100–1106.

National Institute of Mental Health (NIMH). www.nimh.nih.gov. Accessed July 2015.

World Health Organization (WHO). www.who.int. Accessed May 2015.

Chapter 1 · What Are Mood Disorders?

American Psychiatric Association (APA). *Diagnostic and Statistical Manual of Mental Disorders (DSM-5).* 5th ed. American Psychiatric Association; 2013.

Barker ED, Copeland W, Maughan B, et al. Relative impact of maternal depression and associated risk factors on offspring psychopathology. *Br J Psychiatry.* 2012;200(2):124–129.

Batten LA, Hernandez M, Pilowsky, DJ, et al. Children of treatment-seeking mothers: A comparison with the sequenced treatment alternatives to relieve depression (STAR*D) child study. *J AM Acad Child Adolesc Psychiatry.* 2012;51(11):1185–1196.

Fava GA, Rafanelli C, Grandi S, et al. Prevention of recurrent depression with cognitive behavioral therapy. *Arch Gen Psych.* 1998;55:816–820.

Martin LA, Neighbors HW, Griffith DM. The experience of symptoms of depression in men vs women: Analysis of the National Comorbidity Survey replication. *JAMA Psychiatry.* 2013;70(10):1100–1106.

Massachusetts General Hospital. MGH Center for Women's Mental Health. www.womensmentalhealth.org. Accessed May 2015.

Nierenberg AA, DeCecco LM. Definitions of antidepressant treatment response, remission, nonresponse, partial response, and other relevant outcomes: a focus on treatment-resistant depression. *J Clin Psychiatry.* 2001;62(suppl 16):5–9.

Pilowsky DJ, Wickramaratne, PJ, Rush AJ, et al. Children of currently depressed mothers: A STAR*D ancillary study. *J Clin Psychiatry.* 2006;67(1):126–136.

Regier DA, Rae DS, Narrow WE, et al. Prevalence of anxiety disorders and their comorbidity with mood and addictive disorders. *Br J Psychiatry Suppl.* 1998;(34):24–28.

Saveanu RV, Nemeroff CB. Etiology of depression: Genetic and environmental factors. *Psych Clin N Am.* 2012;35:51–71.

Schmidt PJ, Ben Dor R, Martinez PE, et al. Effects of estradiol withdrawal on mood in women with past perimenopausal depression: A randomized clinical trial. *JAMA Psychiatry.* 2015 Jul 1;72(7):714–726.

Sichel D, Driscoll JW. *Women's Moods: What Every Woman Must Know about Hormones, the Brain, and Emotional Health.* Quill;1999.

Teasdale JD, Segal ZV, Williams JMG, et al. Prevention of relapse/recurrence in major depression by mindfulness-based cognitive therapy. *J Consulting Clin Psych.* 2000;8(4):615–623.

Trivedi MH, Rush AJ, Wisniewski SR, et al. Evaluation of outcomes with citalopram for depression using measurement-based care in STAR*D: implication for clinical practice. *Am J Psychiatry.* 2006;163(1):28–40.

Weissman MM, Feder A, Pilowsky DJ, et al. Depressed mothers coming to primary care: Maternal reports of problems with their children. *J Affect Disord.* 2004;78(2):93–100.

Yeung A, Feldman G, Fava M. *Self Management of Depression: A Manual for Mental and Primary Care Professionals.* Cambridge University Press; 2010.

Chapter 2 • Signs of Depression to Look For

Alpass FM, Neville S. Loneliness, health and depression in older males. *Aging Ment Health.* 2003;7(3):212–216.

American Foundation for Suicide Prevention (AFSP). www.afsp.org/ preventing-suicide/suicide-warning-signs. Accessed May 2015.

Centers for Disease Control and Prevention (CDC). National Suicide Prevention Lifeline. Suicide: Risk and protective factors. www.cdc .gov/violenceprevention/suicide/riskprotectivefactors. Accessed May 2015.

Centers for Disease Control and Prevention (CDC). www.cdc.gov. Accessed May 2015.

Centers for Disease Control and Prevention (CDC). *Youth Suicide Prevention Programs: A Resource Guide.* Published 1992.

National Institute of Mental Health (NIMH). www.nimh.nih.gov. Accessed July 2015.

National Suicide Prevention Lifeline. Suicide risk factors. www .suicidepreventionlifeline.org. Accessed May 2015.

Chapter 3 • Support and Communication Strategies

Buckman R. *How to Break Bad News: A Guide for Health Care Professionals.* Johns Hopkins University Press; 1992.

Chapter 4 • Helpful Approaches

American Academy of Sleep Medicine. Sleep hygiene. www.sleep education.com/essentials-in-sleep/healthy-sleep-habits. Accessed May 2015.

Beck A, Rush A, Shaw BF, Emery G. *Cognitive Therapy of Depression.* Guilford Press; 1979.

Bodnar LM, Wisner KL. Nutrition and depression: Implications for improving mental health among childbearing-aged women. *Biol Psych.* 2005;58(9):679–685.

Burns D. *Feeling Good: The New Mood Therapy.* HarperCollins; 2009.

Dunn AL, Trivedi MH, Kampert JB, et al. Exercise treatment for depression: Efficacy and dose response. *Am J Prev Med.* 2005;28(1):1–8.

Frank E. Interpersonal and social rhythm therapy: A means of improving depression and preventing relapse in bipolar disorder. *J Clin Psychology: In Session.* 2007;63(5):463–473.

Jacka FN, Pasco JA, Mykletun A, et al. Association of western and traditional diets with depression and anxiety in women. *Am J Psychiatry.* 2010;167(3):305–311.

Kitchener BA, Jorm AF. Mental health first aid training for the public: Evaluation of effects on knowledge, attitudes and helping behavior. *BMR Psychiatry.* 2002;2,10.

Langlands RL, Jorm AF, Kelly CM, Kitchener BA. First aid for depression: A Delphi consensus study with consumers, carers and clinicians. *Journal of Affective Disorders.* 2008;105:157–165.

Mayo Clinic. Mediterranean diet. www.mayoclinic.org/healthy-lifestyle/nutrition-and-healthy-eating/in-depth/mediterranean-diet/art-20047801. Accessed May 2015.

Mead GE, Morley W, Campbell P, et al. Exercise for depression. *Cochrane Database of Systematic Reviews.* 2009;(3):CD004366.

Mental Health First Aid Australia. www.mhfa.com.au. Accessed May 2015.

Noonan SJ. *Managing Your Depression: What You Can Do to Feel Better.* Johns Hopkins University Press; 2013.

Reivich K, Shatte A. *The Resilience Factor.* Broadway Books; 2002.

Rethorst CD, Trivedi MH. Evidence-based recommendations for the prescription of exercise for major depressive disorder. *J Psychiatr Pract.* 2013;19(3):204–212.

Sanchez-Villegas A, Delgado-Rodriguez M, Schlatter AA, et al. Association of the Mediterranean dietary pattern with the incidence of depression: The Seguimiento Universidad de Navarra/University of Navarro follow up. *Arch Gen Psychiatry*. 2009;66(10):1090–1098.

Sheffield A. *How You Can Survive When They're Depressed*. Three Rivers Press; 1998.

Southwick SM, Charney DS. *Resilience: The Science of Mastering Life's Greatest Challenges*. Cambridge University Press; 2012.

Trivedi MH, Greer TL, Grannemann BD, et al. Exercise as an augmentation strategy for treatment of major depression. *J Psychiatr Pract*. 2006;12(4):205–213.

Tsuno N, Besset S, Ritchie K. Sleep and depression. *J Clin Psychiatry*. 2005;66(10):1254–69.

United States Department of Agriculture (USDA). www.choosemyplate.gov. Accessed May 2015.

United States Department of Health and Human Services (HHS). Physical activity guidelines for Americans. Published 2008. www.health.gov/paguidelines. Accessed May 2015.

United States Department of Health and Human Services (HHS) and the United States Department of Agriculture (USDA). Dietary guidelines for Americans 2010. www.dietaryguidelines.gov. Accessed May 2015.

Yeung A, Feldman G, Fava M. *Self Management of Depression: A Manual for Mental and Primary Care Professionals*. Cambridge University Press; 2010.

Chapter 5 · Finding Professional Help

Highet N, Thompson M, McNair B. Identifying depression in a family member: The carers' experience. *Journal of Affective Disorders* 2005;87:25–33.

Sajatovic M, Jenkins JH, Cassidy KA, et al. Medication treatment perceptions, concerns and expectations among depressed individuals with type I bipolar disorder. *Journal of Affective Disorders* 2009;115(3):360–366.

Chapter 6 · What You Can Do Now

American Academy of Sleep Medicine. Sleep hygiene. www.sleep education.com/essentials-in-sleep/healthy-sleep-habits. Accessed May 2015.

American Foundation for Suicide Prevention (AFSP). www.afsp.org/ preventing-suicide/suicide-warning-signs. Accessed May 2015.

Baldwin DS, Papakostas GI. Symptoms of fatigue and sleepiness in major depressive disorder. *J Clin Psychiatry*. 2006 Suppl;67(6): 9–15.

Benson H. *The Relaxation Response*. 2000 rev. ed. Avon; 1975.

Burns D. *Feeling Good: The New Mood Therapy*. HarperCollins; 2009.

Centers for Disease Control and Prevention (CDC). Suicide: Risk and protective factors. www.cdc.gov/violenceprevention/suicide/ riskprotectivefactors. Accessed May 2015.

Kabat-Zinn J. *Wherever You Go, There You Are*. Hyperion; 1994.

National Suicide Prevention Lifeline. Suicide risk factors. www .suicidepreventionlifeline.org. Accessed May 2015.

Noonan SJ. *Managing Your Depression: What You Can Do to Feel Better*. Johns Hopkins University Press; 2013.

United States Department of Agriculture (USDA). SuperTracker. www.supertracker.usda.gov. Accessed May 2015.

United States Department of Agriculture (USDA). www.choose myplate.gov. Accessed May 2015.

United States Health and Human Services (HHS) and the United States Department of Agriculture (USDA). Dietary guidelines for Americans 2010. www.dietaryguidelines.gov. Accessed May 2015.

Chapter 7 · Anticipating Recovery—Skills to Have in Place

American Psychological Association (APA). Resilience guide for parents and teachers. www.apa.org/helpcenter/resilience.aspx. Accessed May 2015.

American Psychological Association (APA). The road to resilience. www.apa.org/helpcenter/road-resilience.aspx. Accessed May 2015.

Catalano D, Wilson L, Chan F, Chiu C. The buffering effect of resilience on depression among individuals with spinal cord injury: A structural equation model. *Rehab Psychology.* 2011;56(3):200–211.

Dunn AL, Trivedi MH, Kampert JB, et al. Exercise treatment for depression: Efficacy and dose response. *Am J Prev Med.* 2005;28(1):1–8.

Haeffel GF, Vargas I. Resilience to depressive symptoms: The buffering effects of enhancing cognitive style and positive life events. *J Behav Ther Exper Psychiatry.* 2011;42(1):13–18.

Mak WWS, Ng ISW, Wong CCY. Resilience: Well-being through the positive cognitive triad. *J Couns Psychology.* 2011;58(4):610–617.

Masten AS. Ordinary magic: Resilience processes in development. *American Psychologist.* 2001;56:227–238.

Mead GE, Morley W, Campbell P, et al. Exercise for depression. *Cochrane Database of Systematic Reviews.* 2009;(3):CD004366

Rethorst CD, Trivedi MH. Evidence-based recommendations for the prescription of exercise for major depressive disorder. *J Psychiatr Pract.* 2013;19(3):204–212.

Southwick SM, Charney DS. *Resilience: The Science of Mastering Life's Greatest Challenges.* Cambridge University Press; 2012.

Stein MB, Campbell-Sills L, Gelernter J. Genetic variation in 5HTTLPR is associated with emotional resilience. *Am J Med Genet B Neuropsychiatr Genet.* 2009;150B(7):900–906.

Trivedi MH, Greer TL, Grannemann BD, et al. Exercise as an augmentation strategy for treatment of major depression. *J Psychiatr Pract.* 2006;12(4):205–213.

Vanderhorst RK, McLaren S. Social relationships as predictors of depression and suicidal ideation in older adults. *Aging Ment Health.* 2005;9(6):517–525.

Wingo AP, Wrenn G, Pelletier T, et al. Moderating effects of resilience on depression in individuals with a history of childhood abuse or trauma exposure. *J Affect Disord.* 2010;126(30):411–414.

Chapter 8 · Caring for the Caregivers

Barker ED, Copeland W, Maughan B, et al. Relative impact of maternal depression and associated risk factors on offspring psychopathology. *Br J Psychiatry.* 2012;200(2):124–129.

Batten LA, Hernandez M, Pilowsky DJ, et al. Children of treatment-seeking mothers: A comparison with the sequenced treatment alternatives to relieve depression (STAR*D) child study. *J AM Acad Child Adolesc Psychiatry.* 2012;51(11):1185–1196.

DePaulo Jr. JR, Horvitz LA. *Understanding Depression: What We Know and What You Can Do about It.* John Wiley and Sons; 2002.

Golant M, Golant S. *What to Do When Someone You Love Is Depressed.* Henry Holt; 1996, 2007.

Pilowsky DJ, Wickramaratne PJ, Rush AJ, et al. Children of currently depressed mothers: A STAR*D ancillary study. *J Clin Psychiatry.* 2006;67(1):126–136.

Rosen LE, Amador XF. *When Someone You Love Is Depressed: How to Help Your Loved One without Losing Yourself.* Simon and Shuster; 1996.

Weissman MM, Feder A, Pilowsky DJ, et al. Depressed mothers coming to primary care: Maternal reports of problems with their children. *J Affect Disord.* 2004;78(2):93–100.

Weissman MM, Wickramaratne P, Pilowsky DJ, et al. Treatment of maternal depression in a medication clinical trial and its effect on children. *Am J Psychiatry.* 2015;172(5):450–459.

Index

.